THE

WITCH'S HERBAL
APOTHECARY

Rituals & Recipes for a Year of Earth Magick and Sacred Medicine Making

Marysia Miernowska

FAIR WINDS

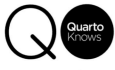

Brimming with creative inspiration, how-to projects, and useful information to enrich your everyday life, Quarto Knows is a favorite destination for those pursuing their interests and passions. Visit our site and dig deeper with our books into your area of interest: Quarto Creates, Quarto Cooks, Quarto Homes, Quarto Lives, Quarto Drives, Quarto Explores, Quarto Gifts, or Quarto Kids.

First Published in 2020 by Fair Winds Press, an imprint of The Quarto Group,
100 Cummings Center, Suite 265-D, Beverly, MA 01915, USA.
T (978) 282-9590 F (978) 283-2742 QuartoKnows.com

Fair Winds Press titles are also available at discount for retail, wholesale, promotional, and bulk purchase. For details, contact the Special Sales Manager by email at specialsales@quarto.com or by mail at The Quarto Group, Attn: Special Sales Manager, 100 Cummings Center, Suite 265-D, Beverly, MA 01915, USA.

24 23 22 21 20   3 4 5

ISBN: 978-1-59233-909-9

Digital edition published in 2020
eISBN: 978-1-63159-784-8

Library of Congress Cataloging-in-Publication Data

Miernowska, Marysia, author.
The witch's herbal apothecary : rituals & recipes for a year of
   earth magick & sacred medicine making / Marysia Miernowska.
9781592339099 (trade paperback) | 9781631597848 (ebook)
1. Witchcraft. 2. Herbs--Miscellanea. 3. Herbs--Therapeutic use.
   4. Formulas, recipes, etc. 5. Magic.
LCC BF1566 .M54 2020 (print) | LCC BF1566 (ebook)
   133.4/3--dc23
LCCN 2019029856 (print) | LCCN 2019029857 (ebook)

Design: Tanya Jacobson, crsld.co
Illustration: Maggie Lochtenberg

Printed in China

For Flora.

You are pure magick.
Divine Love embodied,
wild and free.

I love you.

Mama

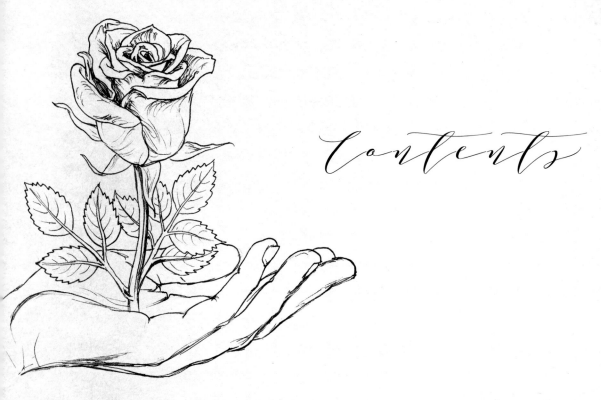

Contents

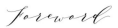

Foreword

Growing up in Ireland, it was difficult to find acknowledgment of these old ways, of the other realms we live alongside and can connect into at will, if we only knew how. For as long as I can remember, magic was always something hidden, shrouded in mystery and only shared with a chosen few, a secret club that was impossible to find, let alone join!

It was rare to find anything other than snippets and whispers of magic or the occasional family cure and recipe that were not easily shared and were often kept secret. Even so, I had always felt they were my ways, listening to plants and their spirits, their medicine, our need to be in service to them in return for the gift of life and healing they offer us.

I had always longed for this book to exist, to guide me, but it only came into being now, through this wonderful gentle soul, Marysia Miernowska, who has generously and openheartedly gifted it to us all, her weaving of the old ways, the green ways, in *The Witch's Herbal Apothecary: Rituals & Recipes for a Year of Earth Magick and Sacred Medicine Making.*

We should all celebrate and honour Marysia for bringing this beautiful tapestry of knowledge into being. For pulling together the healing arts, the magical relationship with nature that most of us have forgotten. It has been too long a broken cord, and it is so important right now to heal our broken relationship with the Earth.

Marysia has demystified the magical and unseen. Within this book, anyone lucky enough to find their way into its pages, is offered a restoration of their own healing power, their own light and truth. I felt such relief reading the openness and simplicity of her carefully woven words explaining such important and ancient knowledge. It is a gift to the world and a generous sharing of her gentle knowledge. It offers the truth of this realm we live in, the magic that has always been there, that we threw off in favour of convenience and mindless consumption.

I know this wonderful book will become a cornerstone for every wild woman, every young curious girl, every lost soul that knows we are living outside of the truth. It will bring you home.

All of you reading this are blessed to have found yourself a copy. It will strengthen your truth and nourish your body and soul. Welcome to the true nature of existence.

It's all just pure magic.

—Mary Reynolds

Founder of the global movement We Are the Ark: Acts of Restorative Kindness to the Earth, author of the bestselling book The Garden Awakening: Designs to Nurture Our Land and Ourselves, *and subject of the 2015 biopic* Dare to Be Wild

how to pray

as if approaching a wild animal, a deer
or a sleeping fox
move quietly
enter with awe
bring flowers, sweet talk
honey, or a blessing smoke
music to call the moon and stars down

lower yourself in the face of beauty bigger
than you can hold

forget your name and open
yourself in pure amazement
praising the billions of beautiful mutations, colored
gases, spirits
rising

sing loud, show some leg
speak like a strong wind
call the spirits to gather close
to hear your heart

raise your hands up
shake the ground
as lightning can wake the earth
ring the bells inside you, and sing
the call to worship.
dance like it's your chance to vibrate the air
and wake the gods

shake every atom, call attention
lure the sky down to earth.

let the tears, your soul,
spill open.

take the 2 year old child that is your mind
to the grandmother of all time
kiss her hand the earth,
her eye of sun, her blood you drink
take off your shoes in her night house.
give up with every cell in your body

Gratitude.

then
in your hands uncurl
your soul's deepest longings

and ask like you would
ask a lover
for sweet touch

open the inner doors
let healing hands of the divine
enter

don't forget
please
and thank you

—Sage L. Maurer,
director & founder of The Gaia School of Healing

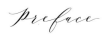

THE BODY FROM WHICH I SHARE

I see us as trees. Marrying the energies of above with below through our bodies, breath, and lives. This book is an expression of the marriage of soil and stars through my vessel. Most of it has come from conversations with plants, listening into silence, dying many deaths, crying at the feet of the Great Mystery, making love through the tips of oak canopies . . . you get the idea. It comes from nonlinear realms.

And yet, by nature, a book is a linear vehicle, hopefully for something vast and wonderful to flower. And so the writing of this has been a translation of energies that exist beyond form, gender, social agreements, and other linear constructs into concepts, archetypes, examples, and practices that are embodied and can therefore move spirit into form. If done well, this can bring medicine to the Earth.

Many ancient mystics have taught that through humans, the energies of the heavens may become manifest in this Earthly plane, and the energies of the Earth may be liberated into the ethers. This book is then made of stars for the soil, plant exhales for the sun. I pray something in it alchemizes with your unique soul, and a ripple of magick moves out of you, becoming liberated as medicine for the whole. But my prayers for this book are many, and I share them later.

The point is, while I am in devotion to the formless, I have a form. While my greatest prayer is for this book to serve the whole, it is written from my being, and my physical being has had a unique experience on this planet. Part of that experience has been informed by my gender, heritage, accent, and other ways I fall into the fabric of our current, limited social and human agreements.

As a female-bodied person, I have traveled through the portals of my female body to connect to Spirit and the Great Mystery. I have gathered tools from these realms, and I share them, aware they do not speak to the entire human experience. While I am evolving in my languaging around gender, I use a system of archetypes in this work associated with a female-bodied experience. I use them, and my body, as portals that connect me to energies beyond gender, time, form, age, and more; nonetheless, I am aware that they have their limitations. I refer to "feminine and masculine" aspects of energy in this work as well, which have nothing to do with gender. I am so glad we are collectively expanding past limitations of defining our forms by gender pronouns and other assumptions. I am a kindergartner in this playground of human word rules. Please forgive any shortcomings in my languaging, and please know that this book is written to all genders, to humans and the nonhuman too.

Marysia Miernowska

The Great Re-Membering

Greetings.

We gather together to remember,
to re-member all parts of ourselves
back into wholeness (*and holiness*).

You are well-come to join me at my fire.

Do you remember that you are made of soil and stars?

Breathe that in and thus weave
the darkness of Earth Mother's flesh,
back into your own.
Inhabit your fullness,
and the knowing in your bones.
Earth my body.

You came here to birth medicine from your inner ocean.
And so, we alchemize plants and prayers
laughter and longing
sunshine and rivers
into potions of healing and love,
bottles of liquid magick catching rainbow light
as the land we love sings songs into the air we breathe.

Together we will create an apothecary.
We will tend your gardens and the wild
with bare feet and open crowns.
Stars and Earth merge through us.
And bubbling like a stream
from the sacred center of our being
flows unconditional love,
a balm for these bodies and times,
replenishing and reviving all thirst
for nourishment and true healing.
Water my blood.

Close your eyes and See.
Make space for the vastness and the void.
We welcome in the Great Mystery.

Together we will ride the currents of air and time.
in the spiral they dance through our lives and
the ancient archetypes
They are threads in the web of galaxies in the night sky.

Travel with me on the Great Wheel
into all directions of what has been and what will be.
We Witches bend the laws of time and space
and arrive more fully
to inhabit the present Now
which ripples into all directions
with each beat of our heart drum.
In the sacred center of our body and being
we weave those who have come before
and those yet unborn.
Air my breath.

Ignite your yes!
Throw tinder in and feed your flame.
Embody your passions
to live through you, as you,
taking form and trans-forming,
thus informing and enlightening
you to who you are. Becoming.

This journey will change you.
In ways born from the fertile void of deepest mystery,
a new spring will awaken as you
blossom and fruit in the summer of You
to harvest the medicine of your gifts for the world
and cut back the dead branches that reach idle.

Together we will feed the Earth once again
as we learn to eat from the table of her belly.
Fire my spirit.

Our circle is cast.
We are in between worlds.
And all that happens in between worlds affects all worlds.

And so it is!

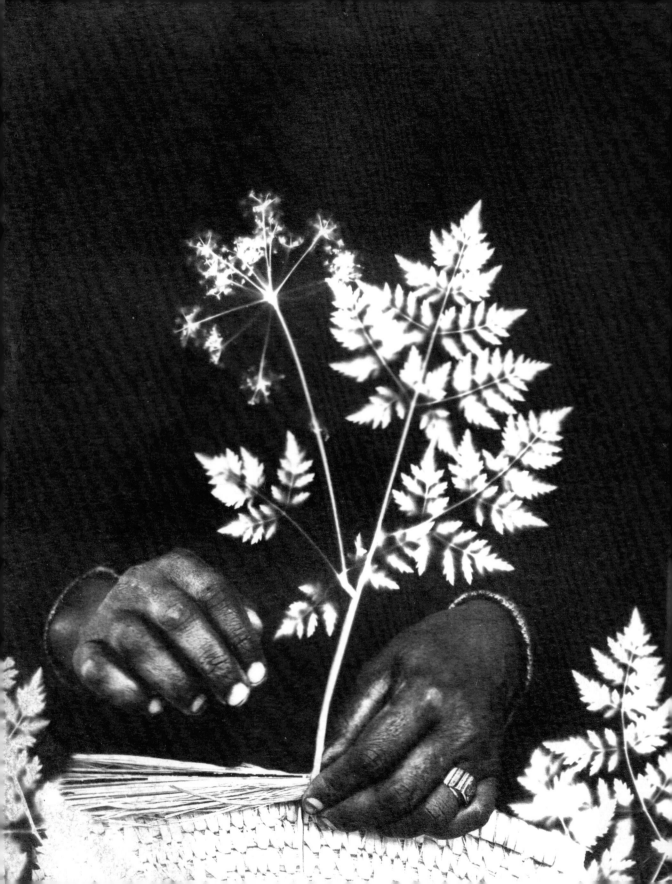

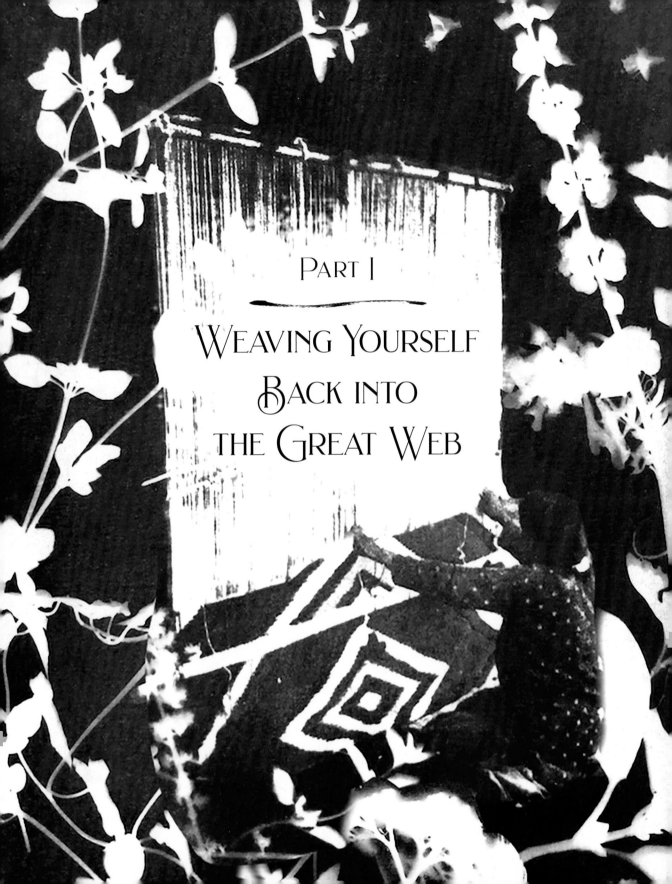

PART I

WEAVING YOURSELF
BACK INTO
the GREAT WEB

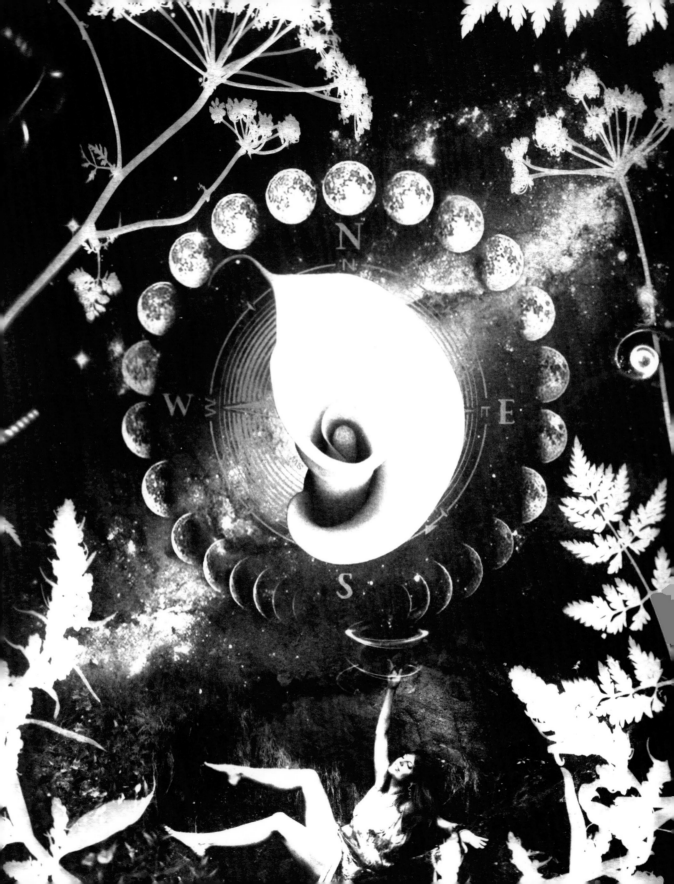

Chapter 1

THE GREAT SPIRAL OF LIFE

How far back do you remember? How have you journeyed to re-member your Self?

Life on this planet has been evolving and transforming itself since the beginning of time as we know it. It is not poetry, but science when I say this: We are descendants of fish that crawled out of the ocean. We breathe air exhaled from trees whose leaves are made of starlight. We have oxygen thanks to the primordial kelps that created this biosphere. The mushrooms we eat come from space; they strengthen both the communications networks in our brains as well as between the plants and the soil. We have stardust in our bones. Our veins echo the patterns of rivers, branches, and root systems. The moon moves the blood in women's wombs to the same rhythm as the tides of oceans.

We are not a part of Nature. We are Nature.

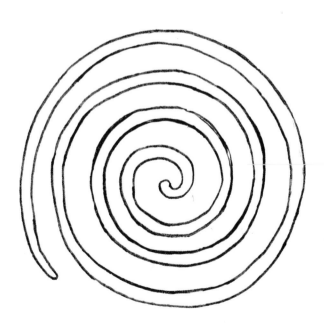

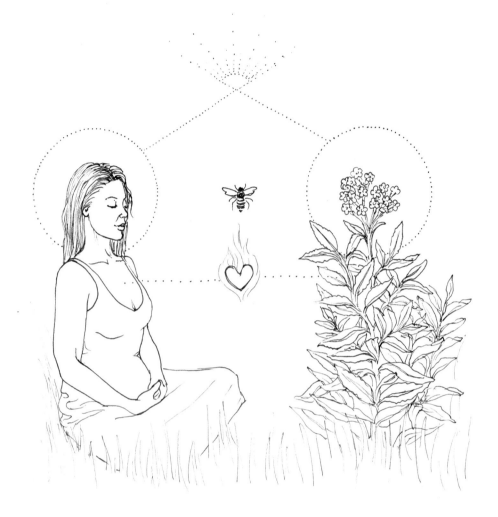

Meet Gaia, Know Thyself

Peoples of all lands and cultures have told stories about how we came to be and why we are here. These tales have connected us, like ancient threads, to the knowings, messages, and guidance of our ancestors. Yet many precious threads have been lost, forgotten, never written, burned, erased, or retold. This book weaves threads of old stories that have come to me from deep listening into silence, from plant and human teachers, from the wind, the night, the stars, wild water, heartbreak, death, renewal, ecstasy, hope, and my own mysterious unfolding, throbbing to the pulse of the Earth's heartbeat as I weave myself deeper and deeper

into the Great Mystery. The story of this work is that of remembering and reclaiming the fullness of our magick and power as part of the Great Web of Life so we can move from heart-centered intention and move out in rightful, healing action. This may be a big dream, but that is why we draw on magick and on our tools as Witches—we who work between realms, affecting all realms, and who bend the laws of time and space to make space for miracles.

Entangled Webs of Our Modern Times

Not very long ago at all, but longer than your short human life, a new story was told. A convincing, cunning, and shining tale that promised riches and ease—oh, how it awoke our human appetite! "Every man has his castle!," the story promised, "and every woman her own appliances! We will be rich like never before!" "There is no need to rely on your neighbors, to share resources, to unite and unionize," the story said. "Follow the ways of this story, and the more you consume, the greater you will be."

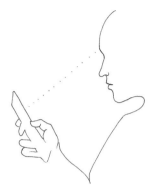

The economic theory of consumerism thus grew into our predominant story since the Industrial Revolution. It asserts that a progressively greater level of consumption is beneficial to the consumer, and it portrays endless growth as something worth striving for. We offered the energy of our imagination and work to the story, which gave it strength and rippled through many voices.

But endless growth is impossible. Every sunrise brings us to sunset. Summer falls to Winter. Human growth and expansion lead to eventual decline and death. A seed becomes a tree, it fruits, it gives food and shade, it fulfills its magnificent role of regulating our biosphere, it experiences relationships with other creatures, and then the energy of its life force begins to wane and return to the darkness of death and renewal.

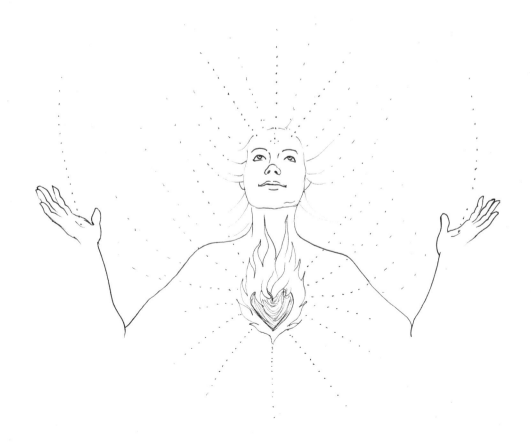

Learning the truths and laws of nature reminds us how to participate in and as Nature—effortlessly blossoming and creating when the time is ripe, or renewing ourselves and retreating into fertile darkness with waning tides. The currents of nature are not a linear path of endless growth—they are cyclical spirals of regeneration. By learning the ways of weaving ourselves into the Great Web of Life, we may ride the regenerative currents of Nature, regenerating ourselves and the world we live in. As Witches, we may use these regenerative ways to experience many cycles of rebirth, death, and renewal in this one human lifetime. The story of regeneration is a love story; it weaves us into something much greater than the story of a small, disconnected human mind. The regenerative currents of nature weave us into the Great Mystery and the Great Web of Life.

The Wheel of the Year

The Wheel of the Year is a visual depiction of the cyclical nature of seasons and time. It is used in many traditions of modern pagan cosmology. The wheel is divided into quadrants, which mark the beginnings of the four seasons and correspond to the four major Earth-worshipping celebrations of the equinoxes and solstices. The four quadrants are each divided again, marking the middle points of the seasons and the "cross-quarter holy days" associated with those moments in time.

Although the wheel itself is a modern depiction, our ancestors of diverse lands and cultures celebrated these sacred moments of the sun's journey of growth and retreat. They celebrated the glory and might of the sun's peak of strength at the Summer Solstice, when the day is the longest of the year, and the holy darkness of the Winter Solstice, when the night is the longest and we pray for the rebirth of the sun. They celebrated the moments of balance at the Spring and Fall Equinoxes, when the days and nights are of equal length, marking the beginning of waxing and waning cycles in nature.

To an Earth-worshipping pagan, it is clear that many of today's Judeo-Christian holidays are riding a wave of celebration that goes back to pagan festivities. Easter and Passover, for instance, incorporate symbols and practices that are more ancient than Christianity and Judaism. They celebrate the renewal of the Sun/Son, reborn in the Spring.

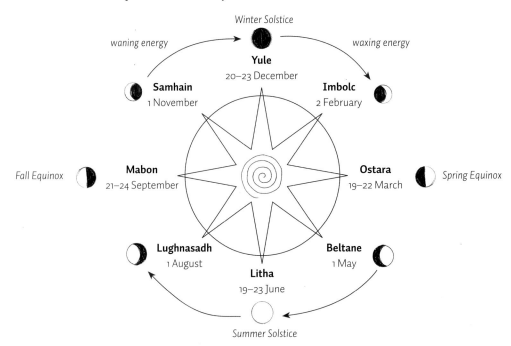

Winter Solstice

waning energy   waxing energy

Yule
20–23 December

Samhain
1 November

Imbolc
2 February

Fall Equinox   **Mabon**
21–24 September

Ostara
19–22 March   Spring Equinox

Lughnasadh
1 August

Beltane
1 May

Litha
19–23 June

Summer Solstice

A Witch is a person who works with the cycles of nature to create transformation and magick. Therefore, we use the sacred moments on the Wheel of the Year as portals to connect to powerful energies of the Earth and Sun. We weave the regenerative currents of Nature's energy into the medicines we make, the rituals we embody, and the offerings with which we feed the land, spirits, our loved ones, and ourselves. This journey we are taking together will offer you rituals and recipes that strengthen your connection to the Wheel of the Year.

Riding the Currents of Nature

Have you ever seen a bird stubbornly decide mid-Winter to build a nest and lay eggs? Can you imagine a whale leaving the migratory pattern of warmer waters that allow for life, choosing to defy his pack's ways? Probably not. Nature teaches us the opportune times to launch new projects into the world, to cultivate growth in our life, to slow down, to retreat, to rest, and to go into dreaming.

Our modern culture, however, pushes us onto a more linear path. We are encouraged to move our life force to a rigorous pace, with the same performance and expectations, from 9:00 to 5:00 (or beyond) every day, regardless of the season of the year or our lives. In order to maintain the continual high energy associated with Summer during the rest of the year, working adults often use stimulants such as caffeine and sugar to keep up their performance. People are expected to work long hours, and our culture values productivity over rest and relaxation. No wonder so many people burn out, become depressed, lose motivation and joy, and get sick. We are not taught how to ride the regenerative currents of Nature.

Riding the currents of Nature means paying attention to the pattern of the sun and moon, to the seasons, and to the ebb and flow of energy inside and around us. Using the tools outlined in this book, we can weave ourselves

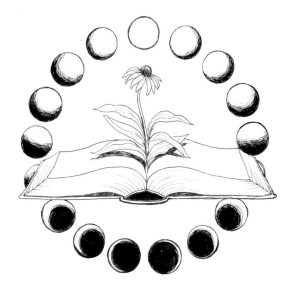

deeper into Gaia. We learn how to move energy that is greater than our own—the energy of the Earth—through our bodies, actions, medicines, and creations. We ride the currents of Nature by following the waning and waxing energies that open in the portals of the Wheel of the Year. However, our journey never brings us to the same point twice, because we move forward on the axis of time. Thus we learn that healing is a spiral dance, as is all transformation and magick.

The Regenerative Way

The regenerative way honors all moments as sacred, important, and part of the wholeness of life. In our gardens, we follow principles of regenerative farming and biodynamic methods. We focus on growing fertile soil and supporting biodiverse ecosystems. We return to pre-industrial farming methods, through which we inherited intact ecosystems and healthy land to grow food in. We learn from our gardens, listen to the plants, pray with the Earth, support life, observe, study, and correct our ways. We weave natural, traditional, time-tested methods that create life in the land we tend. We compost, plant according to the lunar calendar, and

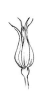
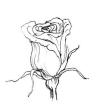
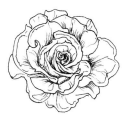
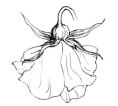
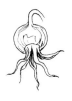

create closed-loop permaculture systems that do not require external inputs, such as fertilizers and other limited resources. We stop tilling soil and pulling weeds, allowing biology to thrive in the fertile darkness below our feet. By increasing organic matter in our soil, we replenish groundwater, feed the small water cycle, and sequester carbon. These regenerative farming methods bring balance and have been shown to help reverse climate change.

In our apothecary, we make medicine regeneratively—that is, as much as possible from plants we grow and gardens we tend and pray in. We practice ethical and sacred harvesting methods to ensure we are benefitting the ecosystems with which we are in reciprocal relationships. We share the medicine we make generously, learning from Gaia herself about the economy of generosity that creates more life and feeds wholeness. We pray into our medicine, weaving in our intentions, learning from the plants and our bodies, sharing from our own experience, and treasuring our sacred plant allies. In the receiving of the bodies, spirits, secrets, and teachings of plants, we give our devotion and are forever asking how we can be of service as the needs of the plants and planet change.

How to Use This Book

This book teaches you to ride the regenerative currents of Nature in your own living, creative process, medicine making, and healing work, and in deepening your relationships with the Earth, Spirit, and yourself.

I recommend you read this book in order. Part I explains the cosmology we use, the Wheel of the Year, and the various access points for magickal connection. Although Part II is divided into the four portals associated with the seasons, we don't only travel the Wheel of the Year over the course of 365 days. We connect to all points of the wheel with each lunar cycle (every 28 to 31 days), as well as traveling it each day. Therefore, you may want to begin reading the chapter of the season in which you find yourself, but ultimately, all the portals are accessible in certain moments of each day, month, and season, and in the archetypes we embody on the larger wheel of our life.

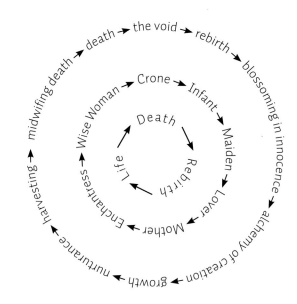

You will notice that many of the practices and rituals are simple. A Witch truly only needs their body, breath, and connection to Spirit to perform rituals of healing, magick, and transformation. Furthermore, a Green Witch draws on their attunement with Nature. Thus, the most important invitation of this work is for you to find your place of union with the Earth. Wherever it is, however it occurs, it is when you feel plugged into the source of chi, the energy of life, the Great Mystery and the magick and love in your heart—it is from that place that magick flows.

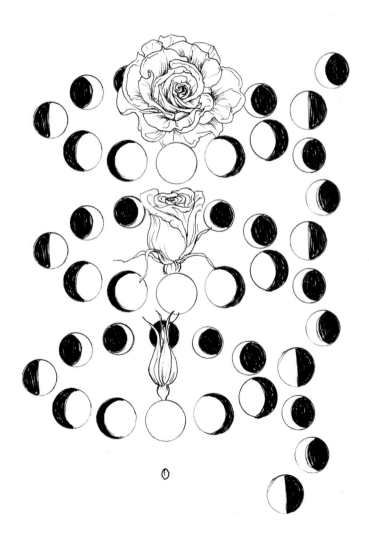

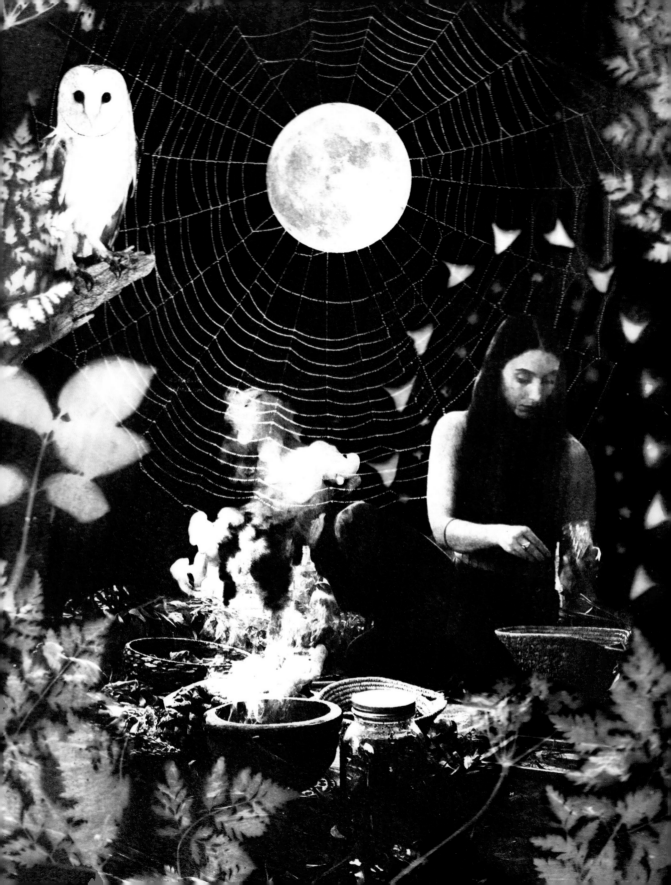

Chapter 2

WHAT IS A WITCH?

Let us reclaim the words Witch *and* magick *and use them as the accessible tools that they are.*

A Witch is an ally and lover of the Earth who works within the cycles of nature. The English word comes from *Wicche, wicce, wicca,* meaning "winer, spinner." Other ethnic names for witches speak of them as those who know, wise ones, prophets, diviners, enchantress, healers, old women, doers or makers, shapeshifters, fateful ones, ancestors, and more. For instance, in Latin, *saga* (wise woman, witch), in Polish, *wiedzma* means "she who sees." In Greek, *pharmakis,* or herbalist; in Irish, *Cailleach,* old woman, sorceress, charmer; in Sami, *noajdisaakka,* or shaman old woman; in Old German, *hagedisse,* or hag, hedge-spirit, wild female being; in Spanish, *bruja,* heathen or pegan.

In English, I associate the word "witch" and *Wicca* to the willow—a medicinal, magickal, and useful tree that connects us to the regenerative cycles of nature. It dies back each fall and rebirths itself, and in doing so it sends rooting hormones that allow other plants to thrive. The willow, like the Witch, knows how to work with the flexibility of reality, how to bend and not break.

Magick is the art of changing consciousness at will, according to Dion Fortune, the British pioneer of modern magick. I also love the definition by earth-based spirituality leader Starhawk: "The art of liberation, the act that releases the mysteries, that ruptures the fabric of our beliefs and lets us look into the heart of deep space where dwell the immeasurable, life-generating powers."

The term *shaman* comes from the Evenki language of Siberia, and it means "the one who knows." We now know that the oldest body of a shaman ever found was female; she lived about twenty-five thousand years ago in what's now the Czech Republic. Archeologists used to assume that notable tombs belonged to men; this reminds us to look beyond "his-story"—the European-centric patriarchal perspective we were taught in school. In our reclamation and remembering, we are invited to discover "her-story," and to bring balance to voices that have been silenced or oppressed.

When training witches, I share that a witch's role is first to master her nervous system. To create magick and healing outside of us, we must begin within. Aware of how powerful our will and intentions are, we must be impeccable with our energy. We seek to know ourselves and master our energy so we do not fall into the traps of unconscious reactions and triggers. We must be able to enter a state of grace at will. From there, the ripples we generate can be medicine.

As we gather the threads of many stories and perspectives, let us enter the realms beyond gender and story. Let us reclaim our inner knowing and step into our birthright as creators of magick, as Witches, as children of the Earth and allies of the Great Mother.

What Is a Green Witch?

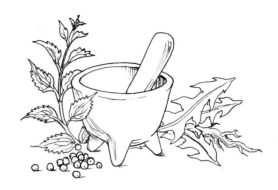

*To be a Witch means that you worship the
Earth as a mother,
and to be a Green Witch means that you heal
the children of the Earth
by bringing them back in
communication Her.*

—Suzan Stone Sierralupe

A Green Witch is a wise one (of any gender) who embodies the Earth as a sacred, living being and aligns with the cycles of nature to create healing, magick, and transformation. She works from her sacred center, which overflows with unconditional love. This state of grace and her practices keep her grounded in the Earth and open to Spirit while she draws on the tools available to her in a wheel of all directions, woven from the tapestry of Nature and mystery. The Green Witch is a healer. Her spiritual practice attunes her heart to the vibration of unconditional love, which is the greatest source of true power on our planet and is the fuel of miracles.

More than anything, a Witch is a devotee of nature. Nature represents the feminine principle, teaching us the regenerative ways that compost systems of oppression and heal cancerous pushes towards perpetual growth. The Witch learns from the Earth Mother how to nourish life, from the wondrous moon how to ebb and flow, and how to work within the one principle that unites Witches, that what you do comes back to you threefold. The craft is nondogmatic, diverse, and has only one rule by which to abide: do no harm.

Plants as Conscious Beings: How to Work with Herbs

When I begin to teach people how to communicate with plants, most think they cannot do it. "Sure, I can see how a shaman can do it, or someone who grew up in the jungle, in an intact culture of natural medicine. But me? A modern person? I won't be able to." Wrong. We can all speak to plants. We can all learn directly from them. It is, in fact, simple. Many of us are already doing it without being aware. Maybe you have reached for ginger at the grocery store and then realized a few days later that you're coming down with a cold and need it. Or perhaps you are struggling with indigestion, so you make yourself a mint tea. In both cases, you are communing with plants. You are drawing on your own embodied experience, on what your body has learned directly from these plants. And you can build on this, in magickal ways.

The reason this is available to all humans is because we and the plants are made of the same elements: air, water, earth, and fire. Getting to know the four elements and how they manifest in our actions, our health, our emotions, our relationships, physical spaces, plants, landscapes, cultures, and so on should be part of a Witch's training. Witches work to create balance, and these are the ingredients we work with on the Earth plane.

However, plants—like humans—are more than the sum of their parts. They have Spirit as well. Green Witches who work with plants as conscious beings develop deep relationships with those we call plant allies. We use our physical senses and the experiences in our body to receive information on how plants affect us and what the alchemy is between us and a medicinal herb. We use our spiritual senses and our presence in meditative states to receive information and healing on the energetic level. After working with a plant for some time, bringing our presence, love, and attention to the relationship, we develop a strong enough connection to call in the spirit of a plant. Some Green Witches, including me, will argue that it is the spirit of the plant that does the healing. That is why herbal medicine made in prayer, calling in the spirit of the plant, is much more potent and effective than mass-manufactured herbal medicine, in my experience. Some traditional folk healers and shamans will work with only one or two plant allies spiritually. They know them so intimately that they have received the plant spirit's song, and in singing it, they can heal people of a huge range of physical, spiritual, and mental complaints—sometimes without using the plant physically at all. May we remember that it is not the number of plants we call allies that makes us effective herbalists, it is the depth of connection that heals.

Learning Directly from Plants: How to Meditate with Herbal Teas

Meditating with an herbal infusion is the core practice taught at the Gaia School of Healing and Earth Education. Sage Maurer founded this herbal school in Vermont in 2001 and has trained thousands of folk herbalists and Green Witches, including me. In 2014, I opened the California chapter of the Gaia School to continue to guide people of all backgrounds in learning how to communicate directly with plants.

The following meditation practice is based on what I learned from Sage Maurer and has evolved as guided by the plants. It is a framework for how you can meditate with plants, thereby connecting to their spirits, receiving deep healing, and opening yourself to their language.

1. Prepare a "simple," an infusion of one herb (see page 55). Choose a plant you wish to get to know, one that calls you. Follow your intuition or any mysterious signs.

2. Create a sacred space where you will commune with this plant spirit. It should feel peaceful and pleasant, relaxing to your spirit.

3. Use the tools and methods that help you access a meditative state, that assist in shifting consciousness. These may include meditative music, burning copal, or a blessing herb (see pages 30 to 31), breathing deeply into your belly, and/or grounding yourself.

4. Call in the directions (pages 27 to 28 have a prayer you can use) and connect to your intention. Call in your guides and any benevolent spirits that can assist in communion, and cast a circle (page 27).

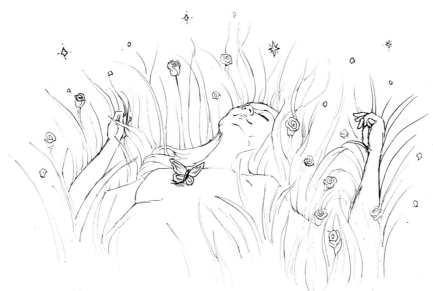

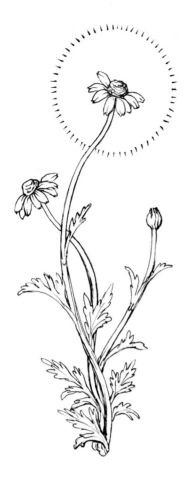

5. Pour your infusion, sit in a comfortable position (I prefer directly on the Earth), and close your eyes. Take some breaths, holding the cup of tea. Arrive in this moment. Breathe. You will keep your eyes closed until the end of this practice.

6. Once you feel calm and energetically open to receive the plant, begin to breathe in the smell of the tea. I call this *sharing breath* with the plant. Meditate on the exhalation of the plant being your inbreath. Use your breath to open your body and begin to invite in the spirit of the plant.

7. Physiologically, the plant begins to enter your blood and body through your nasal passages. Spiritually, the spirit of the plant begins to connect to your spirit. Energetically, open your breath and your heart, and bring your body into relaxation with the intention of receiving.

8. Connect to your sense of smell without losing a meditative state. Simply notice how the smell makes you feel. Maybe a memory or a landscape will come to mind. Perhaps yes, perhaps no; either way, keep on going.

9. Breathe into your heart and the presence of your Self. Energetically, offer your full presence to the spirit of the plant. Introduce yourself to the plant, speaking your name, as if you are introducing yourself to an elder or a healer.

10. Speak your intention of communing, exchanging energy, and receiving any healing or messages the plant has to share with you. Offer it as a humble prayer and request from your heart. Ask your body to open to receive this healing plant spirit. Ask the plant spirit to enter you deeply, going to the places most in need of healing.

11. With a grateful heart, begin to slowly sip. Your eyes should remain closed.

12. Sip, eyes closed, and drink. This is your meditation. Spend twenty minutes or more here.

13. Relax into receiving the energy.

14. If your mind begins to wander, bring it to sensations you are experiencing. Notice if you are feeling the energy of the plant going to any part of the body. Notice what it feels like inside of you. Notice what it makes you think of, if thoughts come up. Continue to breathe deeply and give your mind the task of gently welcoming in the spirit of the plant. Say aloud, in the silence of your experience, "Welcome plant spirit. Mmmm. Thank you. Please show me where you are going."

15. Be in sensation and receiving as much as possible. When the mind wants to participate, give it something supportive to do in deepening the connection. For instance, you can ask questions, such as, "What is your medicine for me?" or "What are you here to help me heal?" You can ask for a

message from the plant spirit. Or you can ask it to give you a healing.

16. You can ask to see the spirit of the plant. Allow your imagination to open and notice whether there is a form, color, being, or landscape. Simply allow, observe, and receive. There is no right or wrong answer. What arises comes from the unique connection of two unreplicable beings: you and the plant, in a unique moment.

17. These are all prompts and possible ways for you to connect to the energy of this plant in your body. Most importantly, follow your intuition and notice how this specific plant and you wish to experience each other.

18. End in gratitude for this plant sharing its body and spirit. In the silence of your meditation, speak words of thanks, acknowledging what you have received.

19. Close your meditation by thanking the directions and elements you invited in when casting your circle. Refer to page 29 on opening the sacred container back up.

Every plant meditation is different, though during group plant meditations, elements of a certain plant will often be shared. Some plants ask me to just be in the receiving, and my meditation feels like an energy exchange or reiki without any visuals or words. Other times, I am taken on a shamanic journey. Still others, my heart opens, the grief or worries I am working through pour out, I ask the plant spirit for help and guidance, and I receive deep wisdom. The purpose of this practice is to cultivate a relationship between you and the plant—physically, emotionally, and spiritually. Practice offering the gift of your full presence and uninterrupted time—something all relationships need to grow and thrive.

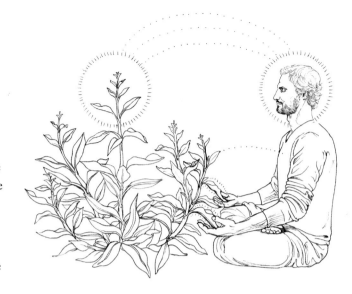

The Wise Woman Tradition of Healing

The Wise Woman tradition of healing is the ancient folk tradition of herbal medicine and traditional healing in which we take root on this journey. Although the term was coined by herbalist Susun Weed, it has long been an unnamed cosmology encompassing folk methods of healing held by elders, midwives, herbalists, grandmothers, wise folk, and shamans, and it can be found crossculturally. It is one of the most unrecorded traditions of healing, and part of its magick is the fact that it moves through invisible webs of nourishment and restoration and away from the spotlight of healing modalities where power and heroism of the healer take center stage. While it is largely unseen, it is foundational to our healing experience as humans.

Practitioners who identify with this tradition heal through nourishment, by supporting others in their transformations, empowering them, and connecting them to the wise one within, *themselves*. This is a non-hierarchical cosmology of healing and regeneration. The power is not in the healer; the power is in the self. "The cure" in the Wise Woman tradition is deep nourishment. We use our bodies to transmit energies of healing, love, and sustenance as we digest those same energies from the Earth that nourishes us.

The wise woman's role is to support transformation in whatever form it takes, including death and disease. Death and disease are not seen as the enemy to be fixed, avoided, fought at all costs. They are seen as vehicles of transformation, messengers, teachers, and, at times, great allies. We are constantly rebirthing ourselves, recreating our world, on both a cellular and spiritual level. There is power and grace in knowing, honoring, and moving within all of the cycles of nature.

This is a woman-centered tradition, though no gender is ever excluded. This tradition is rooted in deep reverence for the energy of the feminine. As herbalist Susun Weed beautifully states, "Female energy is the void of all being: the all-consuming void, the all-birthing void. In the Wise Woman tradition, all health, all coming to wholeness begins with a return to the void."

As an herbalist practicing in the Wise Woman tradition, I work with the plants, their bodies, and their spirits, and I make medicine in sacred space. The strongest feeling I am constantly getting from the plants and the Earth is how infinitely generous they are. We work with plants that are ecologically abundant: wild weeds, "invasives," not rare roots that become endangered as they become a fad. I am continuously, deeply awed by how available this healing is to all of us. The plants of the world want to heal us, to have us eat them, for us to care for them, caress them, give them our love. Plants and people are made to care for one another, to consume one another—we share the intimacy of breath, after all. Every exhale of the plant is our inhale of fresh air; every exhale of ours is their inbreath.

The plants teach us how to care for one another. It is from this place of service to the ones we love, to those who need healing and support, to the plants and the Earth and the spirits, that we magickally create transformation and move toward wholeness and holiness.

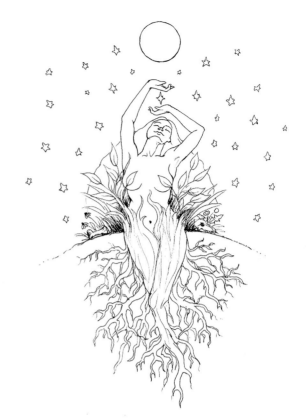

The Elements of Magick

We humans are made of the same elements as the plants, the wind, the stars, and the primordial fire at the center of the Earth. We are woven together in union with the four elements of Earth, air, fire, and water. In my tradition, the four elements correspond to the four directions of North, East, South, and West, respectively. Like the trees that grow by digesting solar rays from the cosmos, bringing harmony to the electromagnetic field of the Earth, we too weave the realms of Above and Below through our bodies, actions, breath, and life. We can draw a sacred wheel around our bodies. The four directions are around us, the fifth is above, the sixth is below, and the seventh is our heart—the sacred center. This is where our inner God consciousness resides, where we vibrate in balance, harmony, and inner peace at the center of the great three-dimensional wheel.

Developing intimate relationships with the seven directions and the four elements is the primary practice of the Witch. It is how we weave our consciousness into the consciousness of the Earth and the Great Mystery.

Casting a Circle

Witches often cast circles before performing a ritual, ceremony, or spell, or when making medicine. The act of calling in the seven directions, the elements, benevolent spirits and guides, and attuning the sacred space with the energy of unconditional divine love, weaves us into the Great Web, protects us, and amplifies the power and magick of our work, while shifting our mind and consciousness so we can move energy from the heart.

The circle may be marked, drawn on the floor, or cast energetically. With no beginning or end, the circle is the perfect container for energy in motion. In circle, we gather as equals, nonhierarchically, and we build energy,

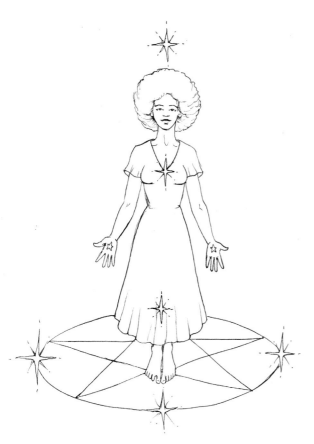

allow it to flow and transform—all within a sacred and safe container. Anything that happens in the circle stays there unless it is released with intention.

There are many ways to cast a circle and create sacred space. Be clear and intentional with your words when calling energies in. Especially when speaking intentions into sacred space, use phrases like "in accordance with divine will" and "if it is for the highest good of all involved." Practice being impeccable with your words and attune the space you create with the power of love.

When I'm teaching or working with a group, we stand in a circle and I call in the directions with my drum, praying to each direction and invoking the elements and benevolent spirits of each direction. Calling in the directions is a prayer cast through the powerful vibration of sound and intention—from the heart and speaking directly to the elements and spirits. Though it may sound poetic, calling in the directions is not about reciting a poem; it is about invoking energies from your praying heart. Upon my calling in each element, my students repeat the closing phrase for each direction together, and with open palms, we rotate clockwise going from East, through the four directions, then to above, then to below, and ending at our hearts in the sacred center. When I am working alone, I usually do not move in a circle but work as the center and cast the circle around me. Following is a prayer you may use or draw on for inspiration to create your own.

Coven Circle Casting

We stand together, fully inhabiting our bodies, rooting through our grounding cords, opening our crowns to the heavens, and breathing into the sacred center of our hearts.

We rub our hands together, opening the energy centers in the palms of our hands, and we face the East.

Spirits of the East, energies of Air, we call you into our sacred circle! With each breath we take, we ask you to

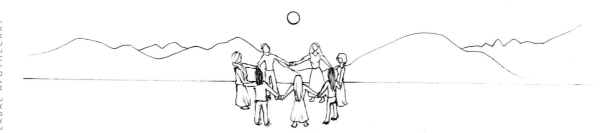

open our hearts and clear our minds, lifting our spirits to the heavens, where we can see the whole from a hawk's perspective. We call in our allies of the East— the winged ones, the sacred smokes, the mountain tops, winds, vines that reach to the sky in trust and wild, spiraling abandon.

And together we say: "Spirits of the East, energies of Air, we welcome you into our sacred circle!"

(Breathe them in.)

Spirits of the South, energies of Fire, we call you into our sacred circle! We ask you to activate and awaken each cell in our being. Empower us as vessels of transformation, so we can burn away all that hinders our highest growth and purest expression. May we rise like a phoenix from our fertile ashes, motivated and ignited in passion and devotion, unapologetically shining our unique light and generously sharing our gifts with the world!

And together we say: "Spirits of the South, energies of Fire, we welcome you into our sacred circle!"

(Breathe them in.)

Spirits of the West, energies of Water, we call you into our sacred circle! Fill our inner oceans with your profound mystery so we may access the depths of our intuition. We pray for all rivers and streams to run wild and free, and for compassion and love to flow unrestrained, honoring the sacred ocean from which all life came. We call in the thunderclouds, the cleansing rain, rivers of renewal, our syblings the fish, whales, dolphins, and flowers that bloom in the light of the moon. Soften us, open our emotional body, and let us be renewers of life.

And together we say: "Spirits of the West, energies of Water, we welcome you into our sacred circle!"

(Breathe them in.)

Spirits of the North, energies of Earth, we call you into our sacred circle! Plant allies, tree teachers, wild weeds, stone, soil, funghi, and green healers, we welcome and honor you. We call in the plant spirits and soul of this land on which we stand. May we arrive as stewards, caretakers, and students, walking gently, our bare feet kissing the Earth. May the plant spirits guide us, heal us, and weave us deeper into the great web of life, so our presence nourishes the Earth, our Mother.

And together we say: "Spirits of the North, energies of Earth, we welcome you into our sacred circle!"

(Breathe them in.)

Spirits of Above, we call you in. We call in the spiraling galaxies, the moon, and the light of the sun that gives us life and energy. We call in our guardian angels and any benevolent spirits who wish to participate in our work and hold this vessel of protection.

And together we say: "Spirits of Above, energies of our guardian angels, the plant spirit, our spirit guides, we welcome you into our sacred circle!"

(Breathe them in.)

Spirits of Below, we call you in. We bow before the layers of memory below our feet, the soil, bedrock, bones, and stones. We honor those who walked this land before us, tending these lands so we can be here today. We welcome the ancestors and ancient ones, may you gather and receive nourishment from our prayers and presence. We invite you to whisper your deep time into our bones, help us remember. We ask for your blessing as we are the ones who are living now, weaving the medicine of that which came before us into the deep presence of this present moment, so there may be life and magick for those yet unborn. Let us be bridges, be with us now.

And together we say: "Spirits of Below, energies of our ancestors, we welcome you into our sacred circle."

Spirits of the Sacred Center, energies of our hearts, we call you in. Divine blossoming hearts, may you open like a summer rose, releasing sweet exhales of pure surrender into the holiest song. May our hearts connect, harmonize to the heartbeat of the Earth, open and become vast like the limitless heavens. We call in our holy plant allies, Tulsi, Rose, Egyptian Blue Lotus, and ask our hearts to be tuned to the song of unconditional love.

And together we say: "Spirits of the Sacred Center, energies of our hearts, we welcome you into our sacred circle."

Our circle is cast.

We are in between worlds.

And all that happens in between worlds affects all worlds.

AND SO IT IS!

Opening the Circle Back Up

Upon completing our rituals, we open the circle we have cast back up and thank all the directions, elemental beings, benevolent spirits, and all that is seen and unseen that came to participate in our work and hold the sacred container.

As we moved clockwise starting in the East, to cast the circle and create a closed, sacred container for magick

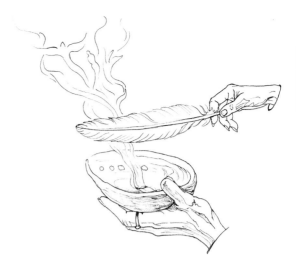

to occur, we then open the space back up, by moving counterclockwise from the North, thanking each direction, releasing and exhaling the energies out and dissolving the container.

> *"May all I say and all I think be in harmony with thee,*
> *God within me, God beyond me,*
> *Maker of the Trees."*
>
> —Chinook prayer

Creating Sacred Space

We create sacred space around us (for ritual, medicine making, prayer, and more) by creating sacred space within us. This begins with shifting our consciousness. Reflect on how you quiet the business of your mind. Notice how deepening and slowing your breath changes the quality of your presence. What helps you arrive more fully into your body? What opens your heart and connects you to the divine?

The practices that bring you into a meditative, open-hearted, shifted state become your tools. Create a ritual that you repeat, thereby training your mind, making it easier and quicker to enter this state. For me, one of these ways occurs the moment I light a charcoal for my blessing herbs—my entire vibration shifts, and

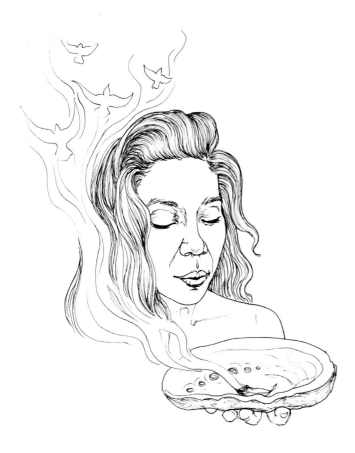

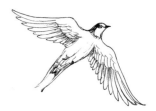

every cell in my body knows that I am going into deep time, into ritual. It is virtually impossible for my mind to start thinking busy thoughts about daily life when I perform this act. This repeated practice has created a new pathway in my mind.

Blessing Herbs, Smudging & Sacred Smoke

Burning sacred resins and aromatic herbs is a simple yet beautiful practice that shifts the energy in space and in our spirits, physically cleanses the air, and weaves our presence and prayers with the spirits of the Earth.

Frankincense, myrrh, copal, palo santo, cedar, and white sage are some of the most recognized ancient sacred smokes currently burned in ceremony and have

been traded around the world for thousands of years. The first three are resins of trees—dried tears of sap that can be placed on a burning charcoal. Each of these crystallized beads of tree sap should be treated with respect and harvested ethically. At the time of this writing, frankinsence, palo santo, and white sage are overharvested. Today, it is disproportionately easy and inexpensive to obtain these herbs. While working with these resins has been a foundational aspect of my training, I now prefer to work with blessing herbs that I have personally, ethically harvested from local plants that are not harmed by sharing their sacred medicine.

Sacred tree resins have been used for thousands of years for spiritual and physical cleansing, or smudging. They have antiseptic and disinfectant properties, and they even boost our immune systems, helping ward off illness. This makes them not only spiritually but physically purifying. It is no surprise that the Three Kings of the Bible are said to have gifted baby Jesus frankincense and myrrh; it would have been a good gift for a baby born in that time—especially in a stable! Any medicine man would be wise to bring this plant medicine to a space that must be purified and to call in angelic protection in for a newborn.

However, when I begin to burn these sacred resins, it is their spiritual properties I immediately feel in my home and heart space. These sacred resins call in the

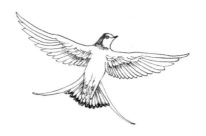

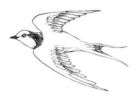

spirits. Each one carries with it a different energy. For me, copal brings in the spirits of our ancestors and of the Earth. It's a sacred resin from Central America, and the spirits of these lands and places awaken when we burn it.

Frankincense has a much higher note, a less smoky and more citrusy aroma. It is my ally for renewing and activating the purity of my home space. With it, my home—my nest and place of refuge, ritual, rest, and renewal—takes on the vibration of my sacred home sanctuary. No wonder frankincense is often burned in churches and sacred sites, the house of God and Spirit.

Over the years of working with sacred smoke and learning about harvesting practices, I have started to work with blessing herbs that I harvest myself. This ensures that the relationship is pure and that I am not causing harm in purchasing these beloved blessing herbs.

One of my favorite resins to work with is pine. It is easy to ethically source your own pine resin because there is an abundance of these trees. When a pine tree's branches are cut or break, it sends the immune system of its sap to heal the wounds. Never take the sap directly from the tree, as it is protecting the wound from infection, and is also sticky and difficult to work with. Rather, run your fingertips around the base of

the tree. You will find little tears that have fallen and dried on the forest floor—these are perfect to receive with prayers and offerings of gratitude (see Sacred Harvesting on pages 34 to 35). And they are not sticky, making them easy to keep.

I also grow my own white sage for harvesting. I teach students never to harvest our beloved *Salvia apiana* in the wild, as it, like frankincense, is overharvested. See more about ethically tending this plant on pages 42 to 43.

Finally, the evergreens juniper and cedar, along with mugwort and other artemisias, make wonderful incense and blessing herbs for burning. These plants are abundant and can be ethically harvested using sacred practices taught in chapter 3.

The herbs that will bring the greatest blessing in the release of their smoke are the ones you have a personal relationship with—those you harvest in prayer, in sacred connection. The plants that have given themselves to you in reciprocity are released in sweet liberation and transmutation when burned into smoke with your prayers for healing.

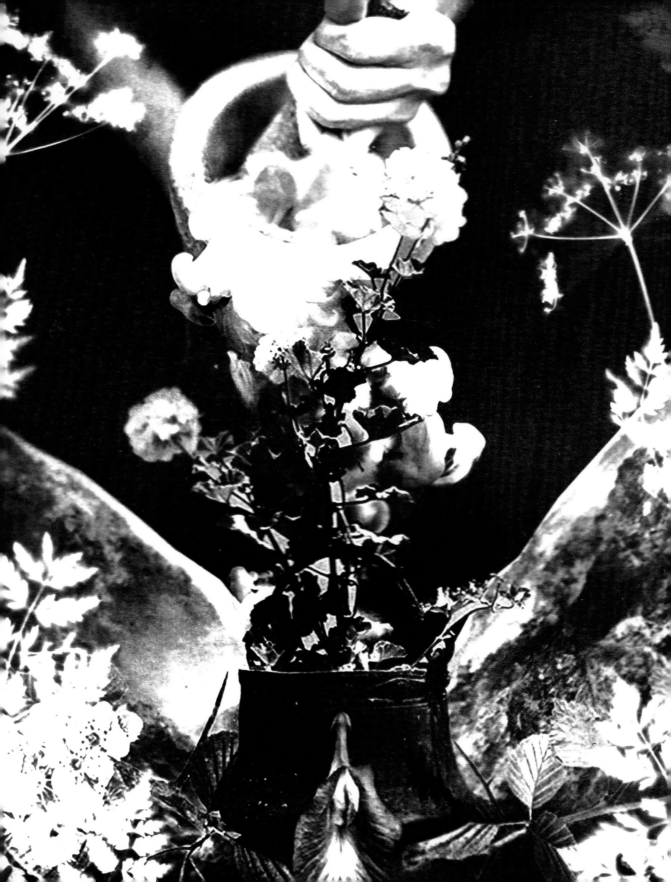

Chapter 3

The Embodied Apothecary & Elements of Magick

To Truly know the world,
Look deeply within your own being;
To truly know yourself,
Take real interest in the world.

—Rudolf Steiner

As we journey through the seasons, the plants in our gardens and in the wild show us how the vital life force energy of the Earth travels from deep Winter roots to freshly birthed leaves in Spring, through ecstatic flowers and ripe, full fruit in Summer, and seeds in Fall that descend back to dream into the fertile darkness of the soil.

As medicine makers, we work with the plants at the peak of their expression to make the most potent medicine, and we learn the language of the plants to know when they are ready, eager to participate, and singing their songs of healing. As we travel through the year together, your apothecary will grow, and you will have medicine for many seasons to come. Focus on building sacred, intimate relationships with the land and plants you love, and they will guide your heart and hands in the making of the most exquisite medicine and healing.

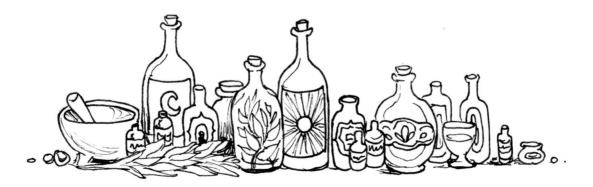

Sacred Harvesting

Sometimes, the harvesting of a plant's physical body feels like the next natural movement we are guided to take in the magickal experience of being in energetic exchange and reciprocal relationship with the plant spirit. Regardless of whether you are taking the body of a plant from your garden or from the wilderness, always follow practices to ensure you are harvesting in harmony, with the agreement and therefore participation of the plant's spirit.

Herbal medicine made in prayer—from harvest to bottle—is energetically and spiritually much more powerful than medicine extracted en masse. You will notice this as you weave your wild heart and prayers into the medicine you make and the land you tend. Crafting your medicine in this way will always touch you deeply and flood you with love and connection. It is medicine that contains not only alkaloids and healing chemical constituents but also the spirit of the plant, the vibration of your prayers, and the magick of your relationship with that place.

When preparing to go harvest, purify yourself; you are going into a sacred exchange and ceremony. For example, you can take a shower with intention, asking the water to wash away any business or chaos, so you can be pure and open to the plants. Or you may smudge yourself with a sacred smoke or resin, cleansing your energetic body with smoke of a plant such as sage, cedar, or copal. It can be as simple as sitting on the Earth, closing your eyes and grounding yourself in your body, placing your hands on your heart, and bringing your awareness into your heart center through prayer, intention, and simple meditation. The grandmothers have taught us never to harvest plants when you are angry, rushed, or in any state other than grateful.

Once connected to the intention and humble gratitude in your heart, take your basket, offering, water, and cutting tools, and go in search of the plant. If you are in the wild, ask the plants that want to be harvested to call out to you. Walk and listen to how you are guided and pulled. If you are visiting a patch of plants you tend in the wild, go as if visiting an old friend, with offerings, joy in your heart, and an openness to greet them anew—without assumptions and with a listening for what messages or requests they have to share.

The Green Witch always asks permission before harvesting. Once, on a beautiful young spring day when living in northern Vermont, I had planned to go harvest nettles and spend the afternoon processing them at home, drying some for later months, and making vinegar and pesto. I had cleared my day. I prepared myself and went, joyfully singing songs, to my favorite nettle patch. When I arrived, I saw my friends green and beautiful, lush and vibrant. My heart flooded with joy, and I sat in my patch, connected to my heart, quieted my self, spoke my intentions and prayers. I made an offering, then cupped my palms around a plant and closed my eyes, casting my request from my heart: "Hello dear friend. It is me, Marysia. I am so happy to be here with you. You look so beautiful and radiant. I would like to make medicine today, vinegar to share with friends to strengthen our bones with your rich minerals, tea so my cells can sing green and pure like you, and pesto! Oh, how I love your pesto! I can't wait to feed my friends and feast on your medicine and love. May I please take some of your leaves and harvest?"

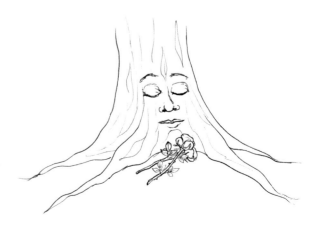

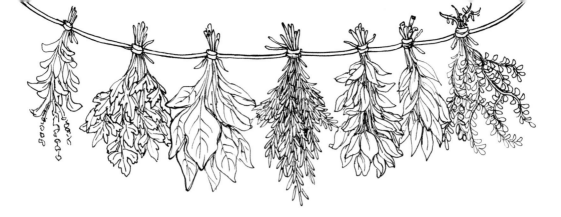

I always felt a joyful "Yes" from this patch, so I was surprised when I heard a gentle, but clear, "No. Not today. Not yet." I honestly felt a little deflated—I had planned my whole day around the processing of nettles. But I listened, of course, gave my love and gratitude for the clear answer, and went home. A couple of weeks later, as I was washing my dishes looking out onto the hills and sunlight, I felt them call from the forest and tug my heart. I took my basket and went out to the woods. There they were, with beautiful fresh strands of green seeds dangling like pearl earrings. They were delighted, and my heart jumped in joy to feel their energy at such a peak state. They said to me, "Now! Harvest us now!" They shared with me that they wanted to make their seeds before I harvested, so I would have medicine with their fresh green spring leaves as well as their potent medicinal green seeds. While previously I had only made medicine with young Spring nettle greens, that year I made a batch of medicine with the seeds as well. It would last for years to come.

Harvest Like a Gardener to Encourage More Growth

Many herbalists are taught that when the medicinal part of the plant is the aerial part (the part exposed to the air) they should cut all the way down to the ground when they harvest it. However, I suggest you harvest as if you are pruning a plant back, so it continues to live and even benefits from a gentle pruning, growing more full and vital. Often, this means I harvest the top third of the plant, which is the most vibrant, cutting back to a nodule, which encourages the plant to bush out and continue growing.

Notice where the energy of the plant is. Follow the wisdom of the seasons in this book. If it is Spring, you are likely to be seeing the chi of the plant expressed as fresh green leaves. Clip some back gently for your use and allow more to grow. If it is Summer, the plant is likely reaching out into the sun and is bigger than it is earlier in the year. The leaves may be drier and less vital if the plant is now moving its energy into the production of flowers.

If you are harvesting flowers, again, make sure there is no visible evidence of your harvesting and that there are plenty of flowers left for bees and the plant itself. You may pinch the flowers back, as in the case of calendula, and then trim the stalks back so the plant does not have to work harder to keep the flowerless stem alive.

In the Fall, we cut plants back so their energy can descend with the Earth's inbreath of Fall and Winter into the dreaming roots. When the aerial part of the plant looks dead, we dig up medicinal roots. Usually, when harvesting the roots of a plant, you will dig up the whole plant. With the exception of comfrey root (see pages 210 to 211), most plants are traumatized if you try to harvest some but not all of the root system. Comfrey thrives when disturbed. It happens to be one of my favorite plant-spirit allies—I call upon it when I myself need to grow new, vital roots after experiencing trauma, a death in myself, or an uprooting.

STEP-BY-STEP SACRED HARVESTING

Take your time as you move through the harvesting process. Relationships are built on offering time, attention, and love, which allow for trust, communion, growth, and magick.

1. Cleanse your energy so you begin with a pure and open heart full of gratitude.

2. Gather an offering, some water, your clippers, a basket, and your journal. For offerings, I keep a gift pouch to which I add special dried flowers and herbs, sacred ash, crystals, shells, or other gifts from nature or remnants of rituals that are meaningful and hold power. In chapter 5, you will find suggestions on how to make your own. If I am ever surprised by an unexpected request to harvest—when hiking, for instance—I will give water if I have a water bottle with me. Plants love the gift of water, especially in the wild. Or I will offer a song or prayer. My grandmother taught me to pull a strand of my hair, and sometimes I weave my hair into plants or wild places.

   As always, use your intuition and let your heart guide you.

3. Go looking for a plant. If you are looking in the wild, make sure there is an abundance of the plant, so harvesting it will not hurt the plant population and ecosystem. If you only see a few plants of this variety, do not harvest it, but do make offerings and share time and energy. Never harvest plants near roads, large paths, or other polluted areas.

4. When you have arrived with the plant you would like to harvest, create sacred space. You may do so by saying a prayer, calling in the directions, burning blessing herbs, or any combination of these things.

5. Introduce yourself to the plant, if you have not met before. If it is a plant from your garden or a patch you tend, greet it like an old friend.

6. Talk to the plant. Share openly, from your heart. Why are you here? Is there something weighing on your heart that wishes to be spoken and released? Are you asking to make medicine for someone in need of healing? Speak out loud (if possible), in whisper, or in the silence of your heart.

7. Speak your intention. If you know what kind of medicine you will make, tell the plant. If you are not sure, that is okay; tell the plant you would like to make medicine and ask whether it has any suggestions or guidance on how to use it. Some of my best recipes and formulas have come directly from the plants at this moment of listening.

8. Make your offering. We never take without giving; by giving a gift, we honor and remember that we are always in exchange and that we align in reciprocity, to create balance and build healthy relationships. I bring a generous pinch of the mixture in my gift pouch to my lips and whisper prayers for the plant to thrive and be fed by my presence and participation. I ask for forgiveness for any carelessness on my part, and I ask for the plant to feel my love and nourishment and that of my fellow humans. I often bring the offerings to my heart and womb before sprinkling them at the base of the plant or burying them.

9. Ask permission. I close my eyes, breathe into my heart and body, breathe into my belly and the flesh sitting on the Earth, and breathe into my feet. I cup my palms around the plant or press my third eye against it and speak to it, asking permission. I wait to feel a yes or a no. Always listen to the plants, because you are building relationships of trust on behalf of all humans.

10. Harvest with an open, grateful, and listening heart.

11. Harvest like a gardener, not a consumer. See page 35 for more on that.

12. Harvest in such a way that no one can tell a human came to harvest. Move throughout the patch, listening to your intuition and trimming the plant back here and there, rather than taking out a bunch in one area and leaving a "bald spot." A general rule of thumb is to never harvest more than 10 percent of the plant or patch. Consider animals or insects who may have a relationship to this patch or plant.

13. Harvest until you feel a message of "enough." Never take more than you will need.

14. By harvesting medicine, you make a commitment to use all the plant material and let none of it go to waste. Always keep your promises.

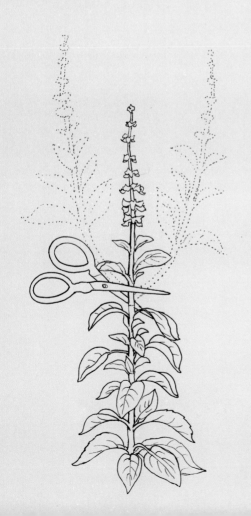

Preparing Your Home Apothecary

Your apothecary will include a magickal and diverse collection of alchemical creations, made as the portals of seasons open and align with your garden, heart, intentions, and the wild land you love.

You do not need many tools, but some are important.

Glass jars. We make our medicine in these, so save old jars and reuse them. Do not use plastic.

A sprouting lid or wide-mouthed tea strainer. This is incredibly helpful because it fits into wide-mouthed mason jars and allows any jar to become a functional teapot. Alternatively, use another strainer for your herbal infusions.

A nut-mylk bag. This is practical for straining medicine and squeezing out all the liquid, as well as for making nut or seed mylks. A cheesecloth is a much messier alternative.

A dark pantry to store your herbs and herbal medicine away from sunlight. You can store them in glass jars or in the plastic bags they often arrive in when ordered online. If they are in a bag, roll out any air—this will help them keep longer.

Dark-colored dropper bottles (such as dark amber). Once your medicine is ready to be strained, you can put it in these tincture bottles and carry them with you in a purse or have them out on your kitchen counter. The dark bottles protect the medicine from light.

Labels or tape. Always label your medicine! Witches always think they will remember what they made and where, but we often forget. Every label should include:

• Fresh (or) dried (Name of Plant)

• in [menstruum: 80-proof vodka/apple cider vinegar/ raw honey? etc.]

• Made on: [date (include whether it's a full or new moon, an Earth holy day, or any other special information about the intention)], [location]

A harvesting basket. Alternatively, paper bags work just fine. Plastic bags do not work because the plants can wilt and mold quickly.

A drying rack, if you plan on doing a lot of drying of herbs. I like collapsible round drying racks because I can hang them or put them away and store them. They have mesh shelves that protect the plants. Always dry your herbs away from sunlight and in a space that has good airflow. It is romantic and beautiful to hang bundles of herbs in your home, but I do this for decoration only. It is not a practical way to dry them for medicine—dust can collect, and sunlight can damage the herbs if they are hung for too long. If hanging herbs, do so in a dark room with good airflow. Loosely placing herbs in a brown paper bag and shaking it daily is a practical and easy way to dry herbs, especially if traveling. A car is a dry warm place as well—if your herbs are in brown bags, you can use your car like a large dehydrator; they will often dry in one day, and then you can store them appropriately.

A pair of good clippers. They should give you a clean cut so they do not hurt the plants when harvesting.

A pouch for offerings (see Summer recipes, page 130).

Blessing herbs. These are a foundational, sacred tool and practice. (See Winter recipes, pages 30 to 31.)

Prayers. Though an invisible tool, opening sacred space is the way we weave our medicine and apothecary into the Great Web of Life.

Your Body as Apothecary

The apothecary and your body are connected through the plants, your hands, prayers, breath, and the beat of your heart. Your body is one of your most important tools. The fire in our belly is our primordial cauldron, and we tend to our flames so we can transmute energy, situations, and lessons from life.

You cannot affect other worlds if you cannot breathe into other realms.

Breath is a fundamental tool for magick as well as meditation, shifting consciousness, healing, tantra—all practices that move our energy out of our small human bodies and weave us into the Great Web of Life.

Land as a Living Apothecary

Your apothecary is alchemized land, water, moon, and passages of time. Every ingredient in your tinctures, potions, salves, and the like is connected to a place, to people, and to an ecosystem. The menstruums (or liquids used to extract the medicinal properties of a plant) we use to make medicine—apple cider vinegar, vodka, and honey, for example—also are full of their own spirit, land, culture, tradition, the energy of humans, the sacred song of bees, and months of fermenting in dark oak barrels. Therefore, consider including the most special and sacred ingredients. They are like golden threads, weaving together all your creations and potions. Honor where they come from.

Planting your own herbs is a powerful way to weave more magick into the medicine you make. You can tend even a small garden or one on a balcony. If you have no space, start a community garden with friends in someone's backyard and share the responsibility and joy of taking care of it. Or connect to an existing organic farm and ask whether you can work with them in planting some perennial herbs alongside their vegetables. It will be a win-win, helping them with pollinators and soil health.

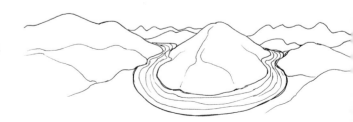

RITUAL OBJECTS:
A LESSON FROM A STONE

One day I found myself deep in the yin energies of winter. It was just days after the Winter Solstice, and I had not gone out for much movement in the fresh air recently, so the energies of both Gaia and my body were yin and slow. I knew I needed to draw in some of the winter sun rays, move my body, awaken my mind, get my heart rate up, and activate my energy. I went outside for a brisk walk with my sister. After a couple of miles, the summit of the nearby mountain called to me. I shot off the trail and bushwhacked up it. Energy began rising in me and around me. Ideas began to flow, inspiration hit, and when I looked down, I saw a rock that, despite being like all the other rocks—a part of this mountain body—called to me.

I picked it up. It fit perfectly in my hand, and I felt how it would be great for ritual.

My blood pumping, my energy body expanding, I felt how easily my energy could be transferred into this stone. It suddenly came to me that all items for ritual become ritual items because we weave ourselves into them. We can do so because we are inherently made of the same stuff.

The ritual items we have been taught to use, such as a cauldron, an abalone shell, or a feather, once arrived in a Witch's arms, and she felt the familiarity that allowed for a transfer. This energy transfers and can continue its transformation outside of the human body of the Witch. It can therefore move beyond the laws of flesh and time.

A shell evokes rituals of cleansing, fertility, water, and our oceanic wombs. The fire in our belly, our passion and purpose, recognizes itself in the flame of the candle. When we hold a wing, our hearts soften in awe of the creature who flew. Our spirits expand, exhaling our prayers, visions, and longings.

The rock spoke to me: "Transfer into my body the energies you are ready to release into eternity. Then throw me into a wild river. I will drown these parts of you, the river will renew and cleanse the energies forever more, and you can go on living lighter, having drowned a part of you in the bottom of the creek."

A WITCH'S TOOLS:
THEY COME TO YOU

A Witch's most important tools are her body, her breath, and a mastery of her nervous system. A Witch draws on her interconnectedness with Spirit and the Earth, and she can thus move great energy and power from realms seen and unseen through herself, creating healing, transformation, and magick inside and then outside of her body in accordance with the one rule, "do no harm."

Some tools, such as the cauldron, broom, wand, pentacle, athame, and chalice, are widely recognized and used, but they aren't necessary for practicing the craft. A Witch gathers tools organically, as she journeys through her life, weaving the magick and the mundane with ribbons of transformation. It is by allowing the tools to come to her serendipitously that they hold power, meaning, and deeper significance. The energy they draw from the Great Web extends beyond her will, intention, and desire. These tools can then be used to help strengthen the power of intention, focus, and embodied energy during ritual.

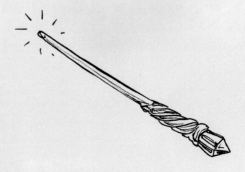

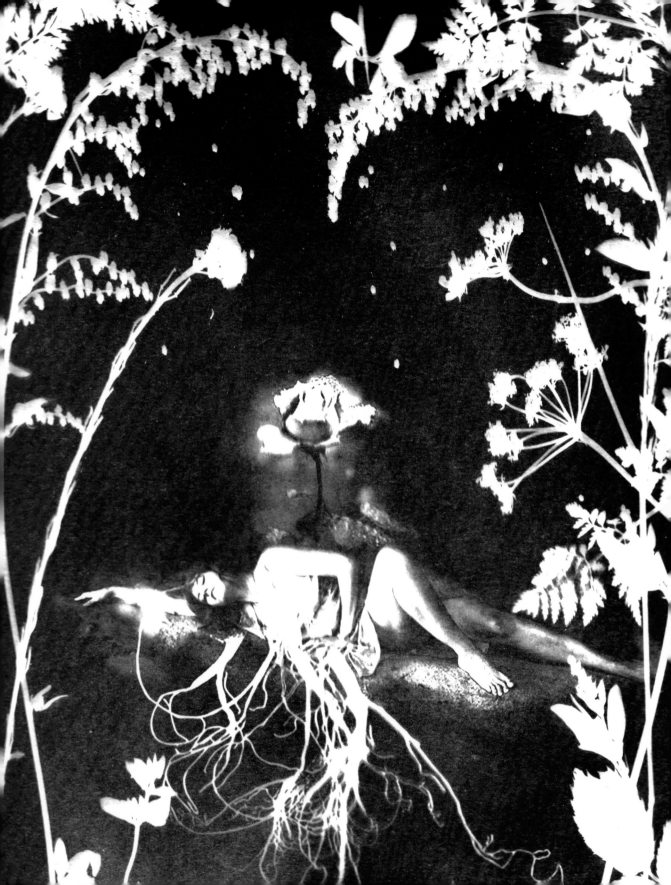

Earth as Lover, Nature as Beloved

Learn to love the land you are in relationship with and allow the Earth to love you back. We have forgotten to love the Earth as Mother, as Lover, and as Child. We have also forgotten to be in a reciprocal, sensual relationship of opening ourselves to be transformed by the touch, love, nourishment, and spirit of the Earth.

Modern humans often dwell in a romantic story of finding the "perfect partner" who will meet all their needs, but it is impossible for one person to fulfill all roles—and anticipating that is a recipe for disaster. It is possible to receive love and support from all directions, seen and unseen, from others and from ourselves. We can love and be loved by humans and nonhumans and find deep nourishment from the love in Nature.

Thanks to my work, I witness the revolutionary healing that takes place when students realize that the spirits of the plants can love them in ways that sometimes humans cannot. I have witnessed countless people who had never received the kind of mothering their spirit desired and were flooded by it in meditation with a plant. Some plants ignite our passion, like the best life coach. Many nurture and heal us like a grandmother, holding us in the healing and unconditional love that is difficult to find in the human realm. Many survivors of sexual abuse I have worked with have found plant allies that awaken their sensuality in a safe way, allowing them to reconnect to pleasure. Still other plants quiet our nervous systems and ground us into our bodies, reminding us that this is a good and safe place to be.

Nature as Beloved: A Practice

Spend a month with the intention of expanding your ability to receive love from non-human realms. (Spring is an ideal time, though any time will do.) In a journal, keep track of experiencing a new aspect of the Beloved in Nature, each day. Let it begin organically—notice if the sun is warming you and it feels good. If so, then let the Sun be your Beloved that day. Spend about fifteen minutes diving into the exchange with the Sun. Greet it as Beloved—yes, actually say, "Why, hello, sun! Sun as Beloved. I welcome you in. Thank you for this warm touch. Mmm, it feels so good . . ." Follow that. Maybe you decide to recline on the grass and gently move your body to receive the sun in different ways. Or perhaps you go under a tree and begin to play with the dappled light on your face as you move. See where it takes you. Replace judgment with curiosity. Play with the Beloved!

Other possible portals through which you can experience the Beloved: warm water in your bath, a flower in your garden, a pet or other animal, the wind, music, art, a tree, a rock, a massage oil, a piece of chocolate, the ocean, a plant spirit meditation, and many more.

Your Garden Is Your Access Point

My garden once told me it was the belly button of the Earth Mother, for me. That there was an invisible umbilical cord that connected me to my garden, and therefore to all the nourishment, magick, and secrets of Gaia. I have found this to be true. And so I tend to my garden as one of my most sacred portals for rituals and one of my teachers of universal truth and mystery. I enter it with bare feet that kiss the ground and fingertips that listen to leaves.

Gardening is a ritual, a prayer. When the plants in my garden begin to pull their chi back into their bodies and their overextended branches begin to get dry and brittle, I enter the garden with my clippers or a sacred knife. I create a ritual of cutting back the places where Summer pushed us into expansion. I reflect on all that I have been doing and committing to in the peak of the

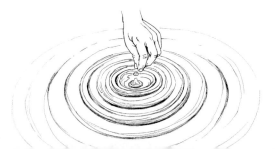

year's solar energy. I use my blade to cut with intention, naming what I will no longer continue doing, so I can deepen in my being. Gardening in a sacred, ritualistic way helps you transform yourself and the world around you. Your garden is part of the Earth's body, the perfect place to pray and speak to the Great Mother.

In all gardens I design, I create a place that is the belly button, the ear, the heartbeat, the access point. My garden has a specific place in it where I pray. I like this space to be large and soft enough to lie down on my belly. Two of the most powerful rituals I use are a release ritual and a burial of burdens, which involve speaking into the Earth. This sacred practice can be used for any purpose and prayer. While it is incredibly healing for releasing grief from the body and burdens, it is also a wonderful way to speak prayers we wish to manifest. Receive the Earth Whisper Ritual on pages 170 to 171.

Tending Wild Places

Get to know wild and untamed land around you.

Aim to build and nurture relationships with two such places this year: one should be in walking distance from your home, such as a place in your yard, a sidewalk strip, an urban park, an empty lot, a park reserve, forest, or intact ecosystem. The other should be a place that calls to your heart and spirit and that is not too far of a drive, so you can visit it at least once a month.

We build relationships with land the same way we do with people. To make a friendship, we must offer what is most precious: our time and our presence. When you make a new friend, you do not project onto them who you think they will be or what kind of a friendship it will become—you arrive, open to experience them, give them your energy, and see what unfolds. It's similar with the Earth. Come without an agenda, simply with an open heart and a dedication to being a good friend. If there is trash, pick it up. Notice the plants and trees

and greet them. Introduce yourself; bring an offering. I ask my students to bring gifts to the land we learn from. Someone dear to me once said, "A true gift hurts a little to give it away. If it doesn't, then it is not a gift, it is something you are getting rid of."

A student, Katie, once made a clay figure of a woman from a local clay she harvested in prayer from land she loved. She clearly put a lot of time and heart into it and gifted it to the dry creek bed where we met to learn from willow. Her love, time, and vision that fruited into her gift dissolved with kind rain and is now woven into the creek bed where the willow grows.

Once you have established a relationship with your two chosen places, it will inspire you to interact with them in new ways. Spend some time observing before doing anything. In permaculture, we observe a piece of land for a year—through all the seasons—before creating anything, garden or otherwise. This reduces the risk of us doing something with the best of intentions that does not actually help the land or use our energy in the best of ways.

You will likely notice certain plants and how they change throughout the seasons, each time you visit. This is some of the best schooling you can receive. Listen for how they call to you to get your attention. You may discover some medicinal herbs, shrubs, mushrooms, or edible weeds in the Spring. If you do, ask them to teach you more about your blossoming friendship. If they offer themselves to you for medicine making, follow the ways of sacred harvesting (pages 36 to 37).

Being a Steward of White Sage

White sage, *Salvia apiana*, is widely used for smudging. It has a long history of use as a ceremonial blessing herb around the globe; though native to North and Central America, it has been traded as far as Asia and Africa for many centuries. The native peoples of Southern California, the land I now call home, have long been stewards of this plant. The Chumash people did not burn white sage in bundles the way some people do now; traditionally, the plant was burned one leaf at a time. The next time you see a bundle, snip it and light one leaf. You will see that you can smudge two or three people—or a whole home—with no more than this. This traditional practice, as well as Native people's regenerative ways of living in reciprocity with nature (read M. Kat Anderson's *Tending the Wild*), kept the plant thriving, in balance.

Today, white sage is overharvested and threatened. People go to places where it is abundant and harvest too much. It has become fashionable in New Age communities to light thick bundles of white sage, wasting so much of this precious plant. As herbalism becomes more popular, consumer culture tries to profit from the commodification of this sacred plant. There is resistance to commodification—recently, petitions have circulated in our community against companies who were packaging "witch kits" with sage bundles, rose quartz, and other "tools" in a plastic box. The appropriation of sacred tools and living plants and stones is deeply offensive, but through education and activism we can work to restore balance and work to heal the harm that has been done.

Living in Southern California, I teach my students never to harvest white sage from the wild. Rather, I encourage them to plant it in their gardens and become stewards of it, teaching people how to use it correctly, speaking up when it is being mistreated, educating others, and working with cultivated white sage. At my apothecary, I sell only cultivated white sage. Unless you are a Native person or have a long-standing and sacred relationship with a patch you have been tending, please do your part to restore balance by planting white sage (it grows as an annual all over the United States and a perennial in Mediterranean climates), burning one leaf at a time, and not buying wild-harvested sage.

What plant can you become the steward of in your ecosystem?

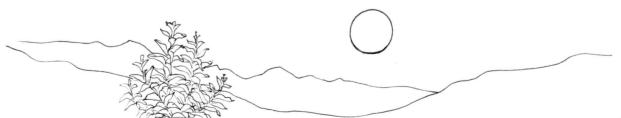

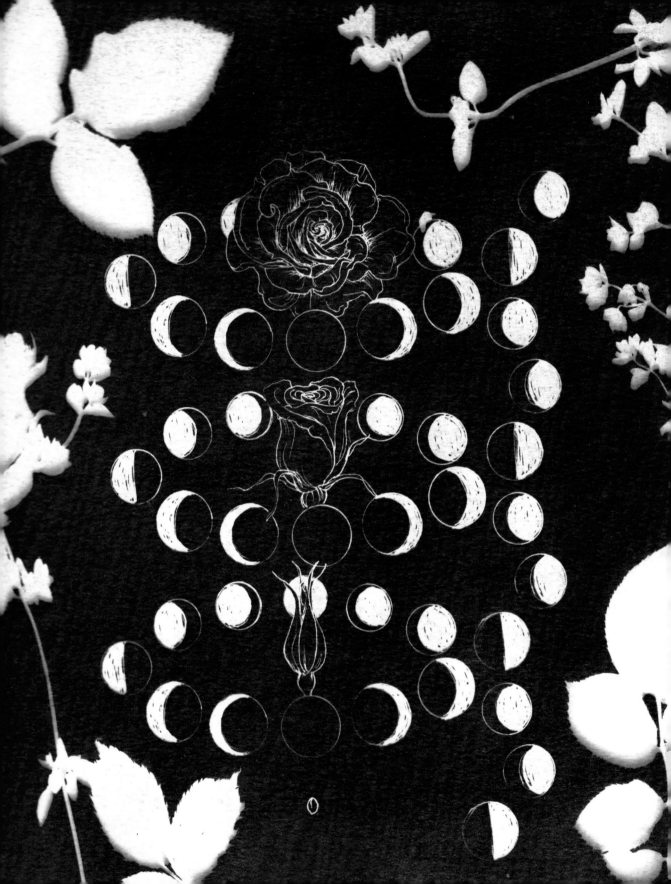

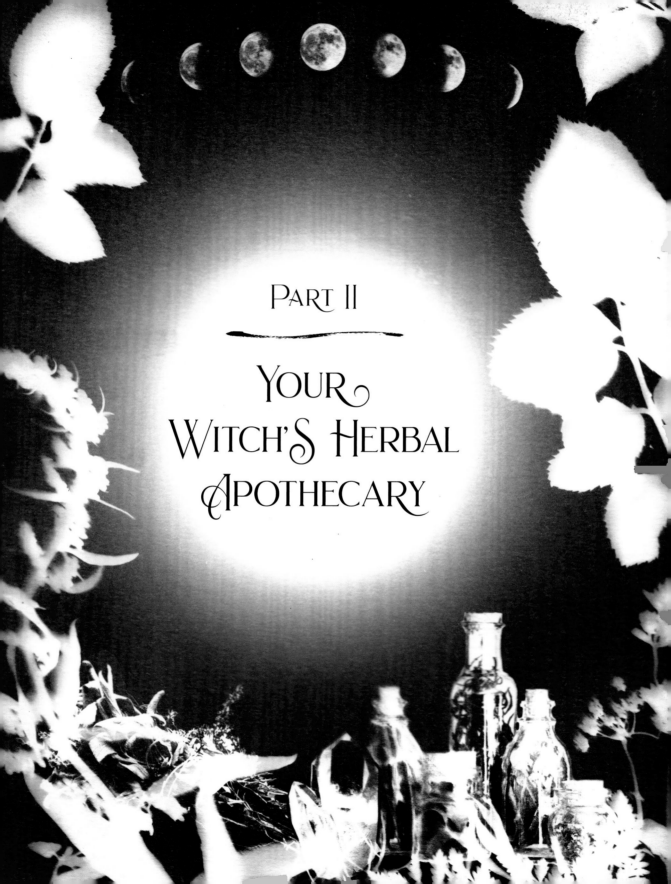

Part II

Your Witch's Herbal Apothecary

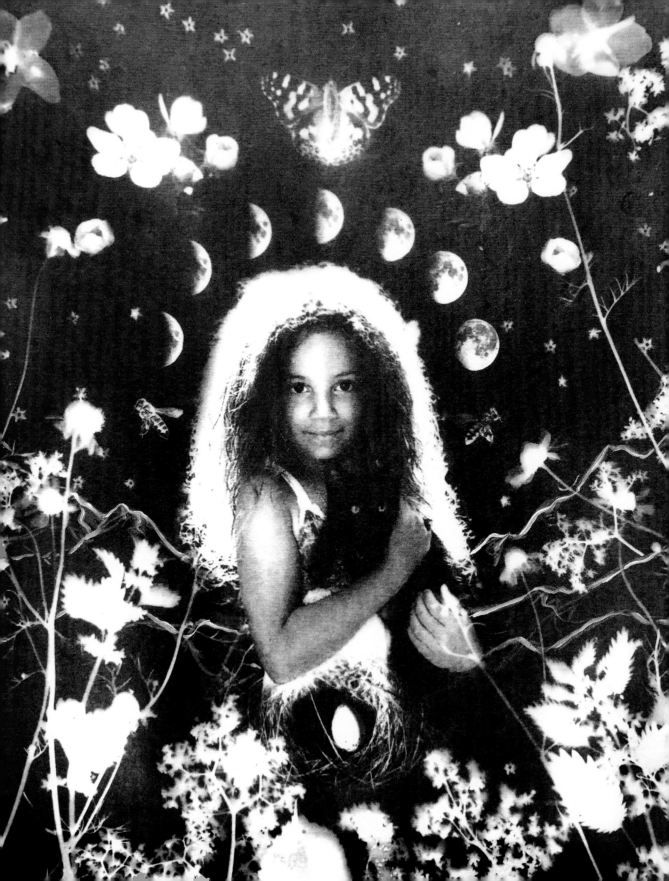

Chapter 4

Earth Magick and Medicine of Spring

Rebirth & Awaken: Ecstasy & Desire | East · Air · The Maiden

The Portal of the East at a Glance

ELEMENT Air

TIME OF DAY Dawn/early morning | 4am–10am

MOON PHASE Waxing

SEASON OF SOLAR YEAR Spring | March, April, May

EARTH HOLY DAYS Ostara (Spring Equinox) | March 19–22; Beltane | May 1

WHEEL OF LIFE ARCHETYPE Maiden | Age 0–21

ENERGIES Waxing, growing, expansive, curious, playful, innocent, delighting, ecstatic, joyful, adventurous, self-oriented, open-minded, mutable, intelligent, fast-moving, transformative, ungrounded, learning, exploring, divination, imagination, visioning

HEALING HERBS

Medicinal weeds and nourishing herbs Nettles, oat straw, dandelion, chickweed, red raspberry leaf, cleavers, burdock, miner's lettuce, violet

Herbal bitters Dandelion, mugwort, blue vervain

Digestive system tonics Lemon Balm; Turmeric; Marshmallow; carminative herbs such as mint, fennel, thyme, oregano, and ginger; and other aromatic and pungent herbs. The nourishing herbs and adaptogens tonify the digestive system as well.

Sacred smokes Mullein, damiana, blue lotus, skullcap, passion vine

Nervines and air balancing plants Lavender, chamomile, motherwort, lemon balm, tulsi, passion vine, skullcap

TENDING THE GARDEN Observing and listening; planning and visioning; planting cover crops; feeding soil with compost; mulching; planting new seeds; planting starts, perennials, fruit trees, and flowers; putting in a medicine garden; planting greens and veggies; harvesting flowers; making flower essences; beekeeping; pruning fruit trees

APOTHECARY Flower essences; wild-harvesting weeds; drying nourishing herbs and spring weeds for tea; making weed vinegars, digestive bitters, blood-building syrups, fresh herbal juices, tinctures, and glycerins; harvesting flowers such as rose and elderflower; harvesting other spring herbs such as yarrow, calendula, and lemon balm

RITUALS Earth Whisper ritual; seeding prayers; rituals with seeds; setting intentions; fertility rituals; pysanky (traditional Eastern European egg painting); rituals of cleansing energy with brooms, eggs, crystals, etc.; purification rituals; herbal bathing; rituals of renewal, (re)birth, and celebration

Gaia Speaks

Awaken, beloved child of mine!
Daughter of the Earth, Son of the Sun.
Open your eyes to the East and greet the rising light.
Let the first rays pierce your mind.
Open your breath
Expand your heart in gratitude . . .
For you are reborn,
each day,
Anew.

Awaken to the throb of life within you,
to the beat of your heart.
Your dreams as seeds in the fertile darkness of
the Great Mystery.

You are young, beloved,
inspired and ready
for the glorious day,
for the ripeness of the year,
for your magnificent life,
which holds more surprises than you could
ever dream of.

Stretch into your sweetness.
Greet your body arising in the morning light
with fresh eyes of admiration and words of welcome.
Each day a new beginning,
each morning the start of spring,
each Spring, the energy of the Maiden,
the innocence of youth
that pulses life into dreams unfolding . . .

Welcome the song of the birds,
the blossoming flowers,
the hum of bees
collecting dripping nectar as I,
the Great Mother, awaken each spring,
oozing my fertile love juices of renewal and rebirth.

Let them wash away the stillness of Winter,
cleansing your inner spaces,
the darkest rooms of your being.
Release the old into my composting flesh.
Be light and free!
Delight in desire and ecstasy!

For the night of the Winter
washes away with the light of dawn.
The cold of the night
melts into softness of a Sun reborn.
The seeds that were planted
penetrate the surface of my soil skin
and you, my child, are
blossoming . . .
becoming . . .
more fully your Self.

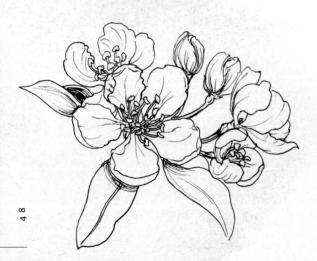

Rebirth to Regenerate Yourself, Expansive Maiden

Spring is the time when all of Nature, ourselves included, is reborn. We reawaken to our purity, our innocence, and the sheer delight of expansive growth so characteristic of children. Tulips, daffodils, and other bulbs that have been dreaming in the darkness of Winter's soil burst through snow, joyfully greeting the young Spring sun. The garden awakens, and Gaia offers fresh wild weeds that cleanse the liver and blood from the stagnation of Winter, regenerating our cells and spirits.

Now is the time to shed the Winter skins of stagnation, old habits, and stale beliefs. As the young Spring sun begins to grow stronger, we encourage the youthful flame inside us and in nature with practices, foods, and rituals.

The archetype of the Maiden corresponds with the Spring portal. Some of the most ancient rituals and holidays celebrated at this time are designed to feed the fertility of the Maiden and the reborn Earth, which ensures our survival and the abundance of full gardens we will enjoy in the Summer months.

All stages between embryo and fertile Maiden have something to teach us about riding the waves of regeneration and cultivating the growing life force of the Spring months. Thus, we honor and tend to the medicine and magick of the newborn and child archetypes as well. We renew ourselves by connecting to sheer delight, spontaneous play, and childlike joy.

By playing, we learn. By expanding ourselves through adventure like the youth, we grow and come to know ourselves better, widening our perspective and becoming more open, flexible, skilled, and, ultimately, wise. By renewing our innocence, we can avoid carrying old wounds and blockages into the future, and we can experience a Spring revival in our relationships, creativity, and work. By mothering our inner child and giving ourselves opportunities to play, we can mature from a place of fullness and wholeness without becoming resentful when the responsibilities of the Summer portal demand our energy.

As we delight in the renewal within and around us, we greet the first weeds of Spring and the nourishing herbs in the garden and in the wild. Dandelion, chickweed, wild mustard, nettles, and burdock awaken our wild spirits, cleanse stagnation from our blood and organs of elimination, wake up our digestion, help us in rebirth, and are full of nutrients, minerals, vitamins, and enzymes that flood our body with wild nutrition and a surge of green energy.

In your medicine garden, your perennial herbs will begin to sprout new life. You will be excited to start new seeds and feed the awakening vitality of your soil with compost or a cover crop. Fruit trees will blossom, and flowers will sing to your expanding spirit. It is a wonderful time to make flower essences for your apothecary—a form of vibrational medicine that floods the body and spirit with the resonant frequency of a flower's spirit song.

The East's Portal of Rebirth opens to you each day at dawn, each waxing moon, each Spring season, and in the youth of your life. Use this time to awaken your childlike joy and a sense of play, and to protect your innocence. Support yourself with gentle, nourishing practices and follow your joy and pleasure—they are sacred. The delight in your heart is like the apple blossom, without which there can be no fruit.

Rebirth to regenerate yourself, expansive Maiden.

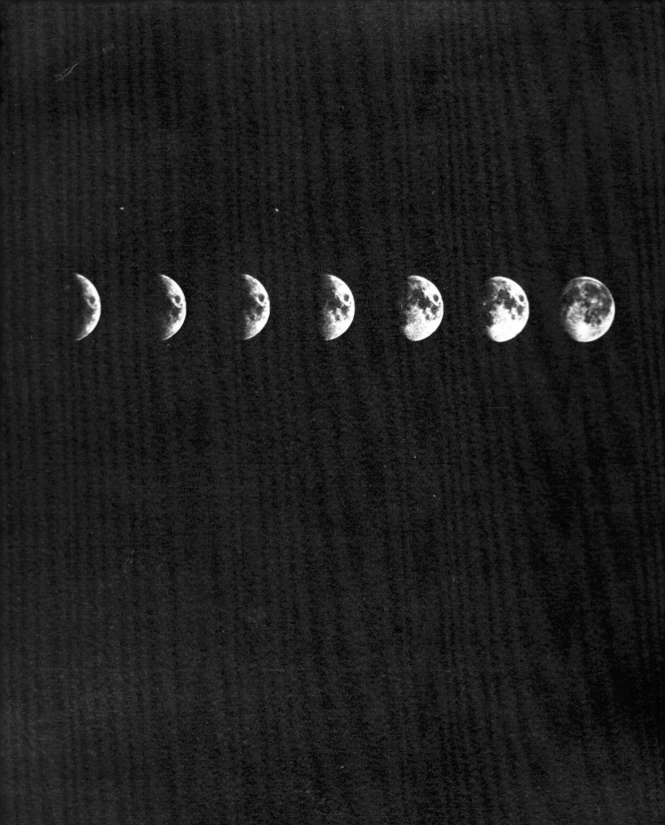

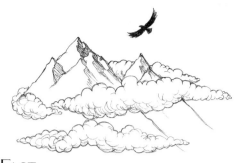

Entering the Portals of the East

The portal of the East is the time of waxing energy present in Nature's cycles. In the twenty-four-hour cycle of a single day, we enter this portal as the sun prepares to rise and when we wake up each morning.

In the lunar cycle, we connect to this portal with the waxing crescent moon rebirthing herself in the dark night sky. Her growing light inspires us to set new intentions for the "moonth." By weaving the prayers in our hearts into the heavens, we can experience the mysterious germination of the seeds we have planted as we follow her into fullness in the night sky.

On our Wheel of the Year, the season of Spring spans the months of March, April, and May in the Northern Hemisphere, with the Spring Equinox (March 19 to 22) marking the official start of Spring, the year's moment of ecstatic rebirth. At Spring Equinox, we once again hang suspended in a sacred moment of balance between light and dark—between the length of day and night, in a midpoint between the Winter and Summer Solstices. From here on, the energy of the sun continues to grow in strength, light, and power until its peak expression on the longest day of the year: the Summer Solstice (June 19 to 23).

Midway between the Spring Equinox and the Summer Solstice, we celebrate the cross holiday of Beltane (May 1), which carries the energy of the mature and fertile Spring. Ancient and modern Earth-worshipping festivals and celebrations feed the fertility inside of us and inside the Earth, as well as our creativity, so we can continue blossoming into a fruitful Summer. It is at Beltane when the Goddess and God within the Great Web of Life consummate their passion and love for each other. The transformative portals of ecstasy, intimacy, union, passion, love, and bliss open as the light of the sun penetrates the moist, fertile, dark Earth.

In the largest wheel we explore together—our lives—the East corresponds to our youth and the archetype of the Maiden. The strong energy of growth and expansion carries us through the immense transformations from embryo to fertile folk—from the seed felt in Imbolc (February) through the rebirth of Spring and the Maiden who seeks expansion and growth (March), to the mature and fertile ones who jump over the ritual fire of passion at Beltane (May), to the peak of energy expressed at the Summer Solstice's Mother archetype.

This is the time to expand our energy and cultivate our rebirth and growth, planting seeds and intentions and mothering ourselves lovingly into sovereign, joyful, powerful, growing beings of light and love!

"Energy is eternal delight."
—William Blake

Entering the East Each Morning

In the wheel of the day, East corresponds to dawn and early morning, from 4:00 to 10:00 a.m. Many ancient spiritual practices encourage us to wake up before dawn to greet the rising sun. If you feel so moved, try for a few minutes of quiet solitude immediately upon waking, before starting your day. It makes a tremendous difference in the management of stress and the health of the spirit to start your day connecting to your first breaths and moments of awareness.

As you birth your rituals for entering the portal of East, allow it to feel gentle, as if you were midwifing your own birth. Create a soft and nourishing environment in which you can transition from rest to renewal. Connect to the energy of the newborn as you call in simple, gentle rituals that bring clarity and connect you to the purity of your heart for the remainder of the day. For instance, you may light a candle upon waking.

Once you have spent some time in simple, silent wonder, allow the energy of gentle love and connection to ripple out from your heart to your body and take form in a nourishing morning practice. This is wonderful time for a few simple self-care rituals that otherwise are hard to fit into the day. Once everyone is awake and the day picks up its energy, we are on a ride until we begin intentionally unwinding at dusk. By then, we are often tired, and a set of different opportunities for nourishment present themselves.

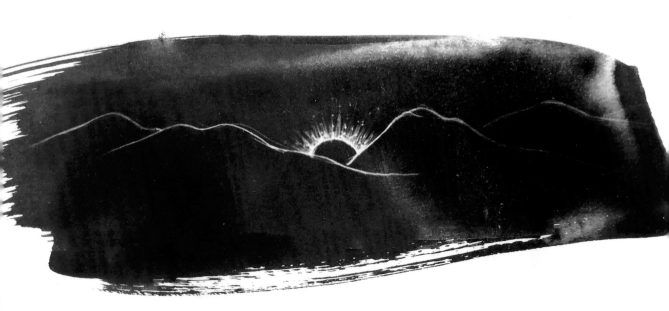

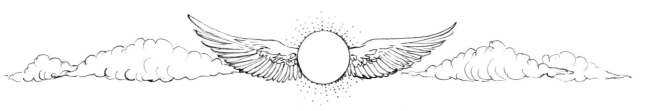

Morning Practices to Weave You into the East

These morning practices are ideal for the Spring portion of the day as well as the Spring times of your menstrual cycle, the lunar cycle, the year, your life, and your children.

- Connect to the feeling of being reborn in the first moments of waking. Let it be very, very simple and sweet.

- Use a gentle alarm sound, such as a birdsong. Compost the habit of reaching for your phone first thing—instead, give your hands a new practice of reaching for your body while still lying in bed. Rest your hands on your belly, heart, or womb and close your eyes, connecting to your first breaths of awareness.

As you breathe, connect to the awareness that you have a living, warm body. I then float in that space between dreaming and wakefulness and recall my dreams. My hands on my belly relax my nervous system so I do not jump into a feeling of rush, but rather enter the day with a calm, slow, sweet, loving energy. I say hello to my body and spirit and give gratitude. In colder months I sometimes stay in bed in this position for my morning meditation; in warmer months I transition to meditate outside in the dawn air.

- Simple self-care morning practices may include tongue scraping, which removes bacteria accumulated overnight.

- Dry brushing your body to awaken your circulation and move lymph.

- Oil pulling, which is wonderful for dental hygiene and is detoxifying to the body.

- Warm abhyanga massage nourishes and calms the nerves for the remainder of the day.

- Drinking warm lemon water or a shot of apple cider vinegar and water upon rising flushes out toxins and awakens the digestive system.

- Drinking an overnight infusion of a nourishing herb on an empty stomach before breakfast.

- Meditation and yoga.

- Greeting the sun with gentle movement, stretching, or song.

- Intuitive dance or a morning dance party.

- Going for a hike or run to energize and activate the body and mind and release stagnant physical and emotional energy.

Everything You Need to Know about Nourishing Herbs

If you incorporate only one practice into your daily life, I offer you the gem of gems: drinking a nourishing wild-weed infusion daily. Nourishing herbs are mostly wild, abundant, nutrient-rich weeds such as nettles, oat straw, dandelion, chickweed, burdock, red clover, cleavers, and red raspberry leaf. Flooding your body with the vitamins, minerals, and enzymes contained in the vitality of weeds that grow in intact, wild ecosystems is life changing. It is the first and primary practice we teach at the Gaia School of Healing and Earth Education, and each year we see students transformed from the inside out thanks to the nourishing herbs.

Nourishing herbs cleanse, renew, and replenish us with wild vitality as they weave us into ancient Earth intelligence and wild remembering. The weeds nourish our cells and our souls. When we begin to drink them, we often find our bodies gulping them down, quenching a thirst we never knew we had, much less knew how to satisfy. Because they come from wild ecosystems, the soil they grow in is full of biological and spiritual information you will not find in cultivated, tilled land.

Spiritually, nourishing herbs replenish us in a way that makes us feel deeply and intimately connected with the Earth Mother. When I drink an overnight infusion of nourishing herbs, all the cells in my body and my soul rejoice, feeling home and whole.

Physically, nourishing herbs are some of the highest sources of vitamins, minerals, and enzymes. They are healing to the gut and digestive system, are alkalizing, and help our body assimilate more nutrients from food.

They support a healthy circulatory system, build blood, and often tonify the heart. They are gently cleansing to the organs and systems of elimination, helping our body detoxify in a healthy, slow, and deep way. They help our body build new tissue and create new healthy cells, and as such they are great allies for pregnant women creating new life and creating more nutrient-rich breast milk. They support the endocrine system, balancing hormones in all stages of our lives, for all genders. Certain herbs are best for specific phases or hormones. They tonify the nervous system, helping us become more resilient to stress, more adaptable, clear minded, balanced emotionally, and heart centered.

Emotionally, nourishing herbs are grounding. Our bodies relax when they are no longer desperate for nutrients and love, and our emotions consequently become more harmonious. As we drink the nourishing herbs, we take in the spirit of wild places and the body of the Earth. We become more resilient to stress and more compassionate toward ourselves and others.

How to Make an Overnight Infusion

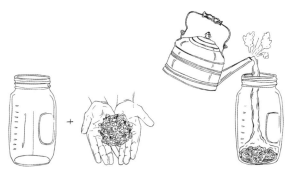
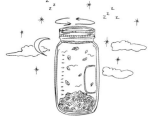
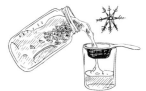

1. Put one handful of herbs into a glass jar.

2. Pour hot water into the jar.

3. Close the lid tightly and let the mixture infuse overnight.

4. Strain. Refrigerate or carry with you.

Drinking these herbs feels like drinking from the teat of the Earth Mother herself. Our bodies relax and energize, and our hearts and minds open. Oh, the miracles that happen when we move through life feeling nourished! We become more joyful, energetic, and inspired. The throb of wildness that the spirits of these plants carry awakens the wild remembering inside of us, giving us fresh vitality and vigor. Drinking wild-weed infusions is the most effective way I know to weave ourselves back into the fabric of the Earth and the Great Web of Life.

Your new ritual is to make an overnight infusion before going to bed each night. Allow it to be your practice. Each night after tidying up the kitchen after dinner, infuse your herbs and leave them out on the kitchen counter so you may effortlessly receive them upon rising in the morning.

Although all nourishing herbs have some healing characteristics in common, each plant also has its own personality and special gifts. The plant profiles that follow will educate you more on each herb. I recommend choosing one and working with it daily for a month, noticing the layers of healing, insights, transformation, and gifts received. After a month you will have developed a strong personal connection to and knowing of this plant, and you may continue working with it daily or switch to another. Mixing nourishing herbs and creating herbal blends works better once you know each one well in your own body. Otherwise, if consuming many herbs at once, you may be unsure which plant is doing what. In our tradition of herbalism, we like to work with "simples"—one herb at a time—so we develop an acute knowing of how this plant's healing manifests. This makes you a better herbalist and, ultimately, will help you formulate better blends.

Spring Nourishment and Cleansing

Our morning practices cleanse us of night stagnation, waking up our bodies with loving intention, breath, and movement. They cleanse toxins and awaken the flame of the digestive system. In the Spring and in the morning, we are given opportunities to cleanse and become light, bright, and energized.

The meal associated with the portal of the East is breakfast—the breaking of the night's fast, thus ending the Winter portion of the wheel of the day. Begin your day with your nourishing herb infusion, drinking as much of it as your body desires. When your body tells you it is hungry, eat breakfast. However, nourishing herbs are so full of nutrition that they often delay hunger. If you are thin, make sure you are nourishing yourself with food. If you are over your natural weight, notice the feeling of becoming full, simply by drinking the herb infusions. As you continue to drink daily infusions of these nourishing herbs, cravings for junk food and stimulants will likely begin to disappear, and you may find that your portion sizes naturally shrink.

Spring can be an ideal time to lose some extra weight that our bodies naturally acquire to stay warm in the stiller months of Winter. I allow my body to wax and wane with the cycles of nature. My body weight fluctuates by a couple of pounds during the moon and my menstrual cycle, and I gain a few extra pounds each Winter. The Wise Woman tradition takes the approach of nourishment and self-love, and we cleanse stagnation without the rigid, harsh, and often punitive approach of "detoxifying." I find the popular detox diets and cleanses to be hard on the physical, emotional, and spiritual body. The strict rules override our intuition. The nervous system often becomes more anxious as it tries to understand the stress the body is experiencing. Many strict cleanses and diets put the body into "starvation mode" and can feel like punishment.

More importantly, these practices do not cultivate a relationship of trust, deep listening, and caring between the body and soul. In a world of "shoulds" and constantly changing templates for the perfect body, look instead to lifelong cultivation of deep listening to natural cues. Listening to your body will heighten its intelligence and ability to communicate what it needs—after all, our bodies are naturally made

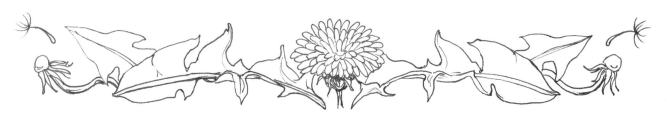

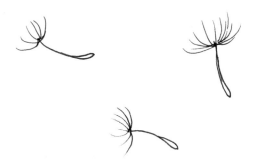

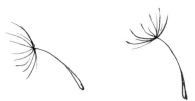

to detoxify. By taking the Wise Woman approach to health, we can lovingly guide the soul into "blissipline" (bliss + discipline) instead of punishment and control. We can allow our bodies to show us what their expression of health looks like, in different moments during our life journey.

That said, Spring is a wonderful time to gently cleanse our body from the inside out. We can easily enhance our body's natural self-cleansing ability, lightening and energizing the body with herbs and supportive practices.

MORNING TONICS

From most gentle/lunar/yin to most energizing/solar/yang.

YIN

- Overnight cold nourishing infusion of nettles
- Overnight hot nourishing infusion of any weeds
- Nourishing herb as hot tea
- Warm lemon water
- Schisandra or rhodiola infusion for caffeine-free energy
- Turmeric golden milk elixir
- Hot raw cacao
- Caffeinated tea or yerba mate
- Matcha
- Coffee

YANG

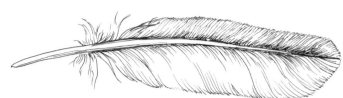

Cleansing in the Spring:
A Nourishing Approach to Losing Winter Weight

Spring is a time to embrace practices and foods that feed our health and renew our bodies after Winter. If that means a little Spring weight loss for you, here are some tips, from most gentle to most actively cleansing.

- Commit to eating what your body is craving when you are hungry, eating slowly and mindfully, enjoying it, and stopping when you are full. *Women, Food and God* by Geneen Roth is an incredible book that teaches us how to transform our relationship with emotional eating through deep spiritual insights.

- The morning body-cleansing practices of tongue scraping, dry body brushing, and oil pulling enhance detoxification, cleansing, and weight loss.

- Drink an herbal bitter twenty minutes before a meal to stimulate the production of digestive enzymes, which help your body break down food. (See page 80 for a recipe.)

- Have fun cooking! Make food with a friend or loved one. Make a meal special and then take your time enjoying it.

- Practice slow, mindful eating. Chew your food to help your body absorb nutrients, to aid in digestion, and to improve energy.

- Practice deep belly breathing before you eat to activate the parasympathetic nervous system and calm the body. If we eat when stressed, we tend to hold weight. Using breath or a nervine tea to get calm before eating makes a huge difference in helping us effortlessly reach our natural weight.

- Drink herbs such as schisandra and gynostemma throughout the day to increase energy while curbing appetite, getting you out of the afternoon slump that can lead to reaching for sweet snacks. Nourishing herbs also decrease appetite. Drink plenty of herbal teas and lemon water throughout the day.

- Drinking yerba mate in the morning delays hunger, increases energy, and stimulates the digestive system. The caffeine in mate and coffee helps with intermittent fasting, though it is taxing on the adrenals. If you are not addicted to caffeine, I recommend you enjoy and preserve your lack of addiction!

- Intermittent fasting is an effective way to lose weight for many people. It prolongs the period at night when we do not take in calories to anywhere from thirteen to sixteen hours; for example, 7:00 p.m. to 11:00 a.m. This changes hormones and helps you burn excess fat. However, it is not effective if you feel starved and then binge eat or eat significantly larger meals. You may drink nourishing herbs, teas, mate, coffee, and so on during your morning fasting to help curb hunger and to keep the body feeling supported and calm. Do your research; this pattern of eating has gained popularity, but it is not for everyone.

- Alternatively, you can try not to eat after a certain time at night, such as 6:00 or 7:00 p.m., without placing a time restriction on the morning meal.

NOURISHING HERB INFUSIONS VERSUS GREEN JUICE

Green juice has gained popularity as an effective way to deliver ample nutrients and minerals directly into the blood, without engaging the digestive system. However, this health fad has a high environmental cost—each glass of green juice takes about 50 gallons (190 liters) of water to produce. And it has a high carbon footprint because the immense amount of pulp goes into landfills, creating methane gas. An overnight infusion of a wild weed such as nettle, oat straw, dandelion, or red clover has more nutrients than most green juices, requires no irrigation or farming footprint, and creates no waste if you compost your herbs or throw them back onto the soil outside.

Furthermore, nourishing wild-weed infusions have more intelligence than their green juice counterparts. The weeds are primordial beings that have adapted through various ecological stressors—and they *thrive*! These herbs have not been bred or modified like commercially farmed plants, so their lineage is ancient. They grow in intact ecosystems, in soil full of microbes and fungi, in a wild web of communication. In contrast, most green juices are made of plants grown hydroponically. These plants are unrooted, growing in plastic containers of water with added chemical nutrient solutions. Drinking nourishing herbs weaves us into ancient intelligent and adaptable wildness that green juices can simply never provide. Replacing your green juices with nourishing herb infusions is better for you and better for the planet.

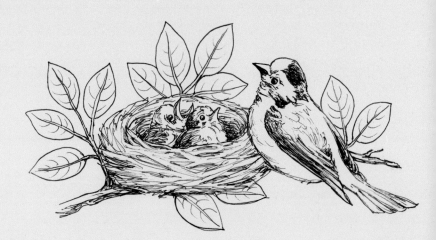

Spring Cleaning

Spring is a time of clearing, cleansing, and making way for the new. Just as we clean our body from the inside out in the morning and in the Spring, we ripple that energy out into the body of our home and lives. A "Spring cleaning" is a powerful spiritual and energetic practice in addition to being practical and physically refreshing.

By digging deep into places in our home where there has been stagnation—boxes, piles of clothes, under the bed, in corners and cabinets—we move dense, stagnated energy and allow it to leave our physical space. As we release the old, we allow for new energy to replace it. We shake out our old identities and create space for transformation, for reinventing ourselves, for inviting in something new.

Feng shui is a Chinese practice developed thousands of years ago to create harmony and health in our environment and lives, using the laws of nature to cultivate more chi, or energy. According to this philosophy, energy must flow in our home, and that means having order and space, even in the hidden places such as in cupboards and under beds.

Go through your possessions. Release anything you do not use and that does not bring you joy. These items are, perhaps subconsciously, weighing you down. Remarkable and surprising spiritual and emotional transformations occur when we radically release possessions. Travel life lighter, with space to be more open.

A Witch will perform the act of Spring cleaning like a ritual, creating sacred space and allowing the physical enactments to connect to deeper intentions. When clearing your home, weave in the magic of the four elements. Use your prayers and intentions to release the old and make room for miracles to blossom in your Self, home, and life.

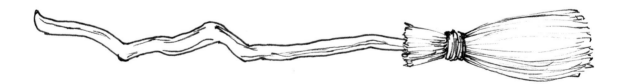

Air

Swing open the windows and the doors, inviting in Spring winds and cool breezes to cleanse your home. Let light pour in. Play music, and let it sing out of the home into the outdoors.

Fire

As you go into deep and dark places to clean your home, burn blessing herbs of local cleansing plants from your garden or ecosystem, such as juniper, sage, mugwort, or cedar or pine resin. These plants have been used for centuries for their physical, energetic, and spiritually cleansing powers. They banish heavy, negative energy from the auric field, and their smoke has antimicrobial and antibacterial properties.

Sometimes, when clearing out an old closet, you may feel flooded by old memories, energies, and a time that no longer exists. Burning sage or another blessing herb helps dispel the energy, allowing it to go back to Source, supporting renewal.

Less commonplace blessing herbs, such as copal, palo santo, and frankincense should be used sparingly, because they are overharvested. I call the resins "tears" to help us remember how precious each drop of tree sap is. Perhaps you will burn a couple of tears of frankincense upon completion of your home cleaning. It has such a high vibration that it can make a space feel like it is vibrating at a sacred, angelic note of light and clarity.

Water

Once the air is fresh and purified and the home is breathing and cleared out, it is time to sweep and wash the surfaces in your home. The Witch's classic magickal tool, the broom, comes in handy for this task. Try sweeping in a counterclockwise direction, calling out all that you are releasing from your home. End by reversing your course; sweep clockwise as you call in new energies and intentions. Wash and purify all the surfaces of your home—the furniture, the walls, and the floor. Standard commercial cleaning products are incredibly toxic and full of by-products from the petroleum industry. Instead, choose a biodegradable product that is safe for animals and children. Or go simple, pure, and cheap by cleaning with white vinegar, baking soda, and liquid castile soap! (See page 80 for an herbal-infused white vinegar for Spring cleaning.)

Earth

Water and feed your plants both inside and outside the home with compost tea, a rich liquid full of microorganisms made from brewing compost. Your resident plants will lift their vibrations and exude aliveness and Spring vitality all around. Sweep the front stoop or porch and tidy up the path leading home. Leave shoes outside the door, as many traditional cultures have always done. Studies show that outdoor shoes worn in the house are a larger source of children's pesticide exposure than eating nonorganic fruits and vegetables.

Finally, bring some of the outdoors into your home. Maybe a branch that needed to be pruned can be brought indoors to blossom and bring in the energy of Spring? Maybe a beautiful river stone or feather you found on a walk would like to come home and be placed on your altar? Fill your home with flowers, sit back, drink some tea, and enjoy the sacred space that is your sanctuary!

May your home be blessed.

May you welcome in the spirits of Nature and find nourishment in your sacred nest.

And now fly, Maiden free, to discover the miracles of all you can be!

CLEANSING AND CHARGING CRYSTALS

I cleanse my crystals about once a month or whenever I am doing a deep cleaning of my space. I usually charge them under the full moon.

Cleanse your crystals by laying them on the Earth outside under the sun and moon for — twenty-four to forty-eight hours. My favorite method of cleansing my crystals is filling a clear glass bowl with ocean water or spring water with sea salt and bathing my crystals in the water and sunlight. This both cleanses them and charges them. Their vibration will be clear, clean, and high when you bring them back home, and if you leave them out under the moonlight or at an important astrological time, such as the Spring of Fall Equinox or a cross-quarter holiday, birthday, or wedding celebration, they will continue to ripple the vibration of that day into your home.

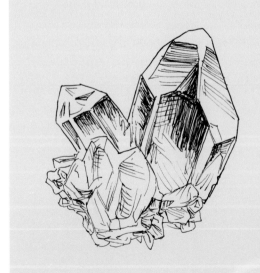

Setting Intentions, Birthing New Life, and Renewing Ourselves

Reborn from the darkness of the new moon, we enter the Spring of all cycles cleansed and open, with visions and hopes for the future. We set new-moon intentions and watch them grow as the moon waxes to full. We cultivate nourishing practices and encouragement to help our metaphorical seeds germinate, connecting to wonder, joy, and delight—energies embodied by children. It is time to be light, carefree, and expansive. Like young people who seek new experiences in order to grow and transform themselves, we too may feel more social, energized, and adventurous following the dark moon.

A woman's time of bleeding is her dark moon and her Winter, and her Spring is the follicular phase of the cycle, which typically lasts until the thirteenth day. It is a time to rebuild blood with herbs such as nettles and angelica. Estrogen increases, the uterine lining thickens, and as Spring matures into Summer, testosterone and libido increase right before ovulation. In order to ride the regenerative currents of menses, one commits to truly resting in their Winter (bleeding) time. Now, in her spring, she feels reborn, energized, motivated, optimistic, and enthusiastic. This is a great time to begin new projects, to follow your own bliss, to take some creative risks, to reach out to others, and to plan the cycle ahead, along with any new intentions or actions you wish to implement. The boldness and optimism of the maiden are best cultivated by having plenty of time to come from the Self. For your own health and vitality and the energy of your creative endeavors, do not shortcut this phase and jump straight into the Summer time of service, taking care of others, and continual action. Stay connected to the delight that will blossom into ripe fruit.

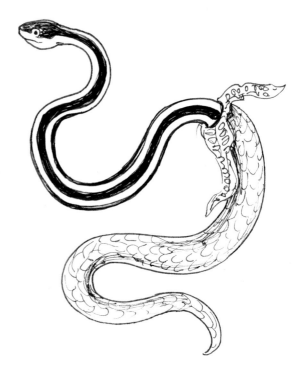

THE MAIDEN ARCHETYPE

The gateway of the East is connected to the Maiden archetype. Here, we connect to the energy of youth that is growing, expanding, and looking for new experiences. We go from the innocence of a child and the need to receive nourishment to the bursting idealism of young adults who seek adventure and experiences that will help them grow and develop. This is a time to broaden our horizons, to learn new things and expand our minds, and to open ourselves to limitless possibilities. This is an important archetype to embody in the creative cycle, and in all journeys on the Great Wheel of Life. There will be a time to refine and focus, but that is not the energy of the East. We must begin by opening ourselves to possibilities we may have not considered, in order to be filled with fresh creative energy, which allows us to birth prolifically time and time again.

The morning practices in this chapter connect you to the embodiment of being reborn anew each morning. Self-care is a priority of the Maiden archetype. Practice to cultivate vigor and optimism as you dream into the possibilities and intentions of your day. The practices of the menstrual cycle, as well as the new moon cycle, encourage us to be a little more "self-centered" than usual in the time that corresponds to the Maiden archetype. For youth to grow into vibrant and powerful adults, it is important for them to follow the beat of their own drum, to follow and discover their bliss. Renew your creative projects and your commitments and responsibilities by connecting to the Maiden archetype in this way as you set new intentions each moon cycle.

And when it is Spring, play! Plan adventures, go outside, move your body in nature, and explore the sun and the breeze as Beloved. Open your senses to the natural world and receive pleasure from connecting to Nature. Lie in a meadow and sing to the sun on your skin. Be wild and free! The joy and delight will bubble into a life-giving spring that will feed you and your loved ones when the time is ripe in the Summer cycles to come.

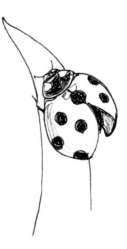

"If a child has been able in his play to give up his whole loving being to the world around him, he will be able, in the serious tasks of later life, to devote himself with confidence and power to the service of the world."

—Rudolf Steiner

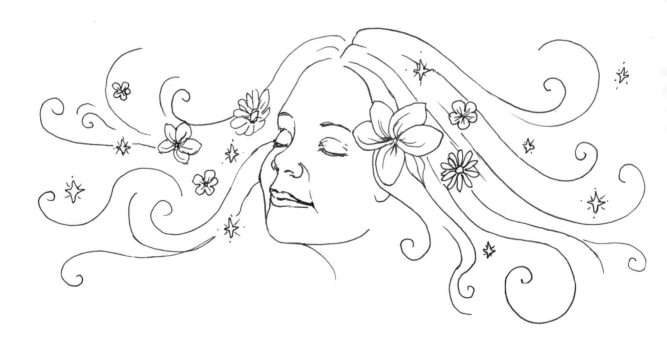

EARTH MEDICINE OF THE EAST: WILD WEEDS

When Gaia's Earth body awakens after the slumber of Winter, she generously offers us medicine and food that is ideally curated for this time in our journey. What are the first plants to pop up in your ecosystem after Winter? Most often they are nourishing weeds—dandelion leaves, chickweed, nettles, raspberry leaves, plantain, miners lettuce, oat straw, and mustard greens.

What do these nutritive plants have in common? They are given to us in absolute abundance by the Earth herself. In the East, we can be like children, receiving the deep nourishment from the Earth Mother, who showers us with prolific edible weeds as if she were encouraging a baby to drink from the breast. This is the time for us to relax into receiving, to flood ourselves with nourishment, so we can be filled with vitality and growth.

The medicinal weeds that are so prolific in the Spring are superfoods. They are high in minerals and vitamins, and they help build our blood. In this way, we see how the plants of Spring are optimal for the corresponding phase of the moon. The blood that was lost during the menstruating time of the dark moon is replenished with our plant allies of the East. Nourishing herbs, the abundant wild nutrition of the Earth Mother, are the foundation of our tradition of folk medicine. Rather than working with rare, expensive plants with ethically questionable environmental sourcing, the Wise Woman tradition works with the plants that are wild, abundant, local, and free. (See more about nourishing herbs on pages 54 to 55.)

Some wild weeds are bitter in flavor. Herbal bitters are wonderful allies for the Spring as well; the taste of bitter stimulates the production of bile in the stomach, aiding us in digestion. When we come into the Spring after a long Winter, we may have excess physical weight or feelings of heaviness, sluggishness, and stagnation. Lucky for us, Mother Nature generously offers us an abundance of food that wakes up our digestion, helps our body naturally cleanse and detoxify, and brings in green vital energy so we too can awaken with all of Gaia in the Spring, during the waxing moon, and each morning. This inner Spring cleaning often feels intuitively right after Winter. Many people will add more fruits and vegetables to release the old and nourish the newness of life. Similarly, starting the day with a nourishing tea will also awaken digestion and nourish our reborn bodies, minds, and spirits.

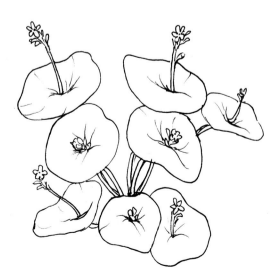

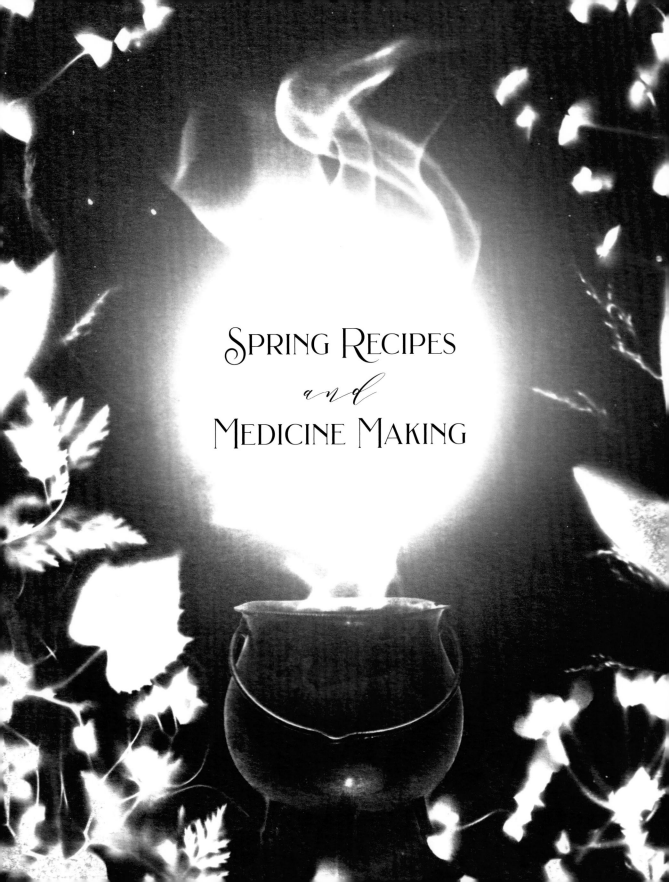

Spring Recipes

and

Medicine Making

Nourishing Herb Tea

Start your day with an overnight infusion of a nourishing herb. This one practice alone will completely transform you. If you have not made an infusion (an extraction of four or more hours), you can still make tea, which is a hot-water extraction of twenty minutes or more. By using more plant material, you can get a strong, deeply nutritive warm beverage. Here is the base method for making it, followed by a couple of my favorite tea blends. Use a quantity of herbs that is roughly what will fit in the palm of your hand. (The folk method is to measure using your own body.)

Yield: approximately 1 quart (946 ml)

> 7 tablespoons (38.9 g) or a handful dried nettles, red clover, oat straw, or a combination

1. Place the dried herbs into a quart jar.

2. Pour boiling water over the herbs and immediately cover the jar with a lid so the medicinal steam does not evaporate. Allow it to infuse as long as possible, or for a minimum of 20 minutes.

. . . .

For nourishing medicinal roots such as burdock or dandelion, extracting the medicine in simmering water leads to a stronger and quicker end product than simply steeping overnight in water from the kettle.

Yield: 1½ quarts (1.4 L)

> 7 tablespoons (49 g) dried nourishing herb root such as dandelion root, burdock root, or eleuthero root

1. Bring the herbs to a boil in 1½ quarts (1.4 L) of water in a small pot, covered, over high heat.

2. Lower the heat and let simmer for 10 minutes.

3. Strain and serve. You can likely reuse the roots again for another extraction.

Nourished and Chill Tea

This crowd-pleasing tea can be served hot or over ice, with or without honey. It's the perfect blend for introducing healing herbs in a delicious and delightful way. It offers the minerals, vitamins, enzymes, and cell-renewal properties of the wild weeds without the earthy taste that we wild Green Witches love and recognize as the delicious taste of the Earth Mother herself—but which can be an acquired taste. The peppermint leaf brightens the blend and gives it a refreshing flavor, making it easy for all to drink, especially children. Adding a spoon of honey makes it absolutely delightful and a favorite for all.

This blend is reviving and renewing while gently cleansing stagnation from the body. It can be an ally for anemics, those who wish to rebuild their blood during or after their moon cycle, and pregnant people who may need assistance with nausea in their first trimester. This blend is grounding to the nervous system and opening to the heart, breath, and mind—it's balancing to the air element. Taken as a daily blend, it may help those who wish to heal their adrenals, to strengthen their nervous system, cardiovascular system, reproductive system, or digestive system, and to balance their mind. As with all nourishing and adaptogenic herbs, the cumulative effect is profound, so I recommend working with this blend every day for a month, a full lunar cycle, or longer.

Yield: approximately 1 quart (946 ml)

> 2 (11 g) tablespoons dried nettles
> 2 tablespoons (11 g) dried oat straw
> 2 tablespoons (3 g) dried peppermint

1. Place all ingredients—or a handful of the blend—in a quart-sized mason jar. Top off with hot water, place the lid on it right away, and let it infuse.

2. Drink after at least 20 minutes as a hot tea, or continue to infuse overnight and drink daily upon rising.

Sweet, Spicy, Alive, and Awake Tea

Working daily with the nourishing herbs to flood the body with nutrients while strengthening the systems of elimination can feel like a grounding, warming, delicious hug, especially when working with the roots of wild weeds and adaptogenic herbs. Nourishing our root chakras is part of our primary practices as Green Witches, and this tea blend builds upon the work of the Winter portal and the grounding and warming "Sweetly Rooted I Rise Tea" found in that chapter (page 201).

Now that Spring is here, we seek to support our activation while continuing to deeply nourish our nervous system so we do not go into a chaotic air element. It's an easy pitfall that feels like a burnout or overwhelm in the excitement of Spring and often corresponds with a body shutdown involving allergies, tiredness, or a cold.

Working with this blend daily could help strengthen your nervous system, immune system, circulatory system, digestive system, and endocrine system and build your deep reserves of energy, while drawing on the stimulating and energizing effects of the adaptogenic herbs.

If you find yourself reaching for stimulants such as sweets and coffee, opt for this blend first. Feel free to add coconut cream and a low-glycemic sweetener for a delicious, energizing, chai-like caffeine-free tonic that gives the comfort, warmth, and energy we seek from coffee.

I keep a pot of this tea on my stove and enjoy it often on chilly days and after a meal as a digestive and to satisfy a sweet craving. With carminative herbs such as fennel and cinnamon, it assists with bloating and digestion as well as circulation, keeping us warm and supporting the heart.

Yield: approximately 1 cup (105 g)

> 2 tablespoons (14 g) eleuthero root
> 1 tablespoon (7 g) burdock root
> 1 tablespoon (7 g) dandelion root
> 2 tablespoons (14 g) astragalus root
> 2 tablespoons (14 g) rhodiola root
> 2 tablespoons (14 g) marshmallow root
> 3 tablespoons (11.3 g) Ceylon cinnamon chips
> 2 tablespoons (12 g) fennel seeds
> 1 slice (½ teaspoon worth) turkey tail or reishi mushroom (optional)
> ½ teaspoon (4 g) licorice root
> ½ teaspoon (4 g) ginger root

1. Combine all ingredients and store in an airtight container.

2. Use one handful of the blend per quart (946 ml) of water. Either make a hot overnight infusion or simmer gently, covered, on the stove for at least 30 minutes. Add more water as necessary.

Black Herbal Coffee

For better or worse, I have become a connoisseur of single-origin, fair-trade organic coffee. My love of coffee—and of my adrenals—has made me determined to meet my need for coffee's comfort and energy in herbal ways that do not push and deplete my nervous system. If you have a need for a boost of energy, consider matcha, cacao, or mate beverages, which have caffeine, or working with rhodiola or schisandra, two stimulating adaptogens.

To satisfy my desire for the delicious flavor of coffee, I used to work with medicinal mushrooms from my native Poland, but some of them are currently overharvested, so I no longer do. I grieve the overharvesting of my beloved mushrooms, which were some of my closest herbal allies; they completely satisfied and healed my coffee addiction. This recipe is a close second for matching the flavors of coffee. It is grounding, nourishing, and supportive to the nervous system and organs of elimination. It is not stimulating and is caffeine free.

Yield: ½ gallon (1.9 L)

> 1 small slice of turkey tail mushroom (about
>   1 teaspoon worth)
> 3 tablespoons (21 g) roasted dandelion root
> 3 tablespoons (21 g) roasted chicory root
> 2 tablespoons (14 g) burdock root
> 1 tablespoon (7 g) fo-ti root
> 2 tablespoons (14 g) eleuthero root
> 1 tablespoons (7 g) astragalus root
> 1 tablespoon (7 g) marshmallow root
>   (optional)
> 2 tablespoons (7.5 g) Ceylon cinnamon
>   chips (optional)

1. Medicinal mushrooms should be decocted (gently simmered with a lid on) in order to get a strong water extraction. A little sliver of dried or fresh medicinal mushroom will go a long way. Begin this blend by decocting the turkey tail with the cinnamon chips, if using them, in 1 gallon (3.8 L) of water for a couple hours.

2. Turn off the heat and let the mixture cool to about room temperature.

3. Bring the mixture back to a gentle simmer for a couple hours once again. Repeat this throughout the day until about half of the water has been reduced.

4. Add the remaining herbs and bring back to a simmer for 1 hour, making a strong black herbal "coffee." I keep this pot on my stove and heat it up, enjoying many cups of this herbal coffee a day. Pour it into a large jar or container and store overnight in the fridge without straining.

Morning Elixirs

A morning elixir made with adaptogenic herbal powders, healthy fats, and collagen (optional) can replace or accompany breakfast while giving us the protein, fats, and vitamins we need to fuel our bodies and souls. It can be a wonderful midmorning treat that helps us continue rising towards the energetic peak of the day. It can also lift us out of the afternoon slump, satisfying the desire for something sweet, filling, and delicious without bogging down the digestive system or bringing in stimulants such as caffeine or sugar.

How to Build an Epic Elixir

Liquid Base + Herbal Powders + Healthy Fat + Low-Glycemic Sweetener + Fixins = Elixir

Blend all ingredients in a high-speed blender to create a frothy beverage. Sprinkle with optional fixins to serve to yourself or a friend!

LIQUID BASE	HERBAL AND OTHER POWDERS	HEALTHY FAT	LOW-GLYCEMIC SWEETENER (OPTIONAL)	FIXINS (OPTIONAL)
1 mug, serving = 1 cup	½ teaspoon– ½ tablespoon	1–2 tablespoons	1–2 teaspoons	
(Hot) water is always a great option. You can also use tea—an overnight nourishing infusion (page 55) or tea from a teabag, etc. Using an herbal tea base instead of water is a great way to get more medicine in your elixir! Infusing a bag of green tea, Earl Grey, or other caffeinated tea can give your elixir an extra energetic boost. Water plus raw juice, such as pure cherry, carrot, celery, apple, spinach, etc., can add delicious flavor when paired correctly with the herbal powders and can substitute the need for any other sweetener.	Adaptogen and other powders that pair well together include eleuthero, maca, ashwagandha (use sparingly—it's bitter), shatavari, mucuna, fo-ti, dandelion, burdock. Cacao pairs well with these. Make a green blend using spirulina and algae with green herbal powders (e.g., alfafa, nettles). Matcha tea powder Collagen powder has no taste and pairs well with any of the powders above, adding protein to your elixir.	Coconut cream Coconut butter Cacao butter Coconut oil Grass-fed butter Ghee	Monk fruit (zero calories, natural, zero glycemic) Xylitol (zero calorie, low glycemic) Raw honey Coconut sugar Maple syrup Liquid stevia (zero calories, zero glycemic)	Dash of mineral-rich salt, such as Celtic or Himalayan 1 teaspoon Flora Sagrada Rose Hydrosol Sprinkle of ethically sourced bee pollen Sprinkle of rose petals Grated nutmeg Sprinkle of cinnamon powder Sprinkle of raw cacao nibs Dash of cayenne pepper

Light and Bright Blessed Day Morning Elixir

This is an uplifting, feminine twist on a classic golden mylk tumeric elixir. It is rich in adaptogens and minerals, and it's extra nourishing to the sacral chakra, reproductive system, and heart.

Yield: 1 serving

> 1 mug (240 ml) hot water, hot Earl Grey tea, tulsi rose herbal tea, or jasmine infusion with flowers
> ¼ teaspoon (0.5 g) turmeric powder
> ½ teaspoon (2.5 ml) vanilla extract or ¼ (0.85 g) teaspoon vanilla pod seeds
> ½ teaspoon (1 g) maca powder
> ¼ teaspoon (0.5 g) shatavari powder
> ¼ teaspoon (0.5 g) eleuthero powder
> ¼ teaspoon (0.5 g) astragalus powder
> 1 teaspoon (6.5 g) raw honey
> 1 tablespoon (7 g) collagen powder (or pea protein powder for vegetarians and vegans)
> 1 tablespoon (19 g) coconut cream (or replace half of liquid base with hemp or oat mylk)
> For fixins: bee pollen, rose petals

1. Blend all ingredients except fixins in a high-speed blender.

2. Sprinkle with bee pollen and rose petals. Serve immediately.

Comfort Yum Morning Elixir

As the name suggests, this is a delicious, decadent-tasting elixir full of adaptogens and mineral-rich plants. It's a real treat. Enjoy it slowly in full luxuriation and bliss.

Yield: 1 serving

> 1 mug (240 ml) hot water, hot Earl Grey tea, or tulsi rose herbal tea as a base
> ½ teaspoon (2.5 ml) vanilla extract or ¼ teaspoon (0.85 g) vanilla pod seeds
> ½ teaspoon (1 g) maca powder
> ¼ teaspoon (0.5 g) eleuthero powder
> ¼ teaspoon (0.5 g) astragalus powder
> ½ teaspoon (0.5 g) fo-ti powder
> ¼ teaspoon (0.5 g) roasted dandelion root powder
> ¼ teaspoon (0.5 g) mucuna powder
> 1 tablespoon (20 g) maple syrup
> 1 tablespoon (12 g) ghee
> 1 teaspoon (5 g) coconut butter or cacao butter
> 1 tablespoon (5 g) cacao powder (optional)
> 1 tablespoon (5 g) collagen powder (optional, or pea protein powder for vegetarians and vegans)
> For fixins: ground cinnamon, nutmeg

1. Blend all ingredients in a high-speed blender.

2. Sprinkle with cinnamon and grate a little nutmeg on top. Serve immediately.

Collagen Protein Matcha Elixir

This blend is rich in antioxidants, protein, vitamins, minerals, and collagen, making it a beautifying morning breakfast elixir. It is balanced in healthy fats, nutrients, and superfoods, and it can replace a morning meal. The matcha powder adds a nice caffeine boost, and the hemp milk and protein ground us for long-lasting energy into midday.

Yield: 1 mug (240 ml)

> ½ cup (120 ml) hot frothed hemp mylk (for a creamier elixir, use more mylk and less water).
> 1 tablespoon (7 g) grass-fed, organic collagen protein powder (or pea protein powder for vegetarians and vegans)
> ½ tablespoon (3.5 g) matcha tea powder
> ½ tablespoon (3.5 g) maca powder
> ½ tablespoon (3.5 g) spirulina, chlorella powder, or a superfood green powder blend
> 1 teaspoon to 1 tablespoon (weight varies) sweetener of choice (monkfruit, raw honey, coconut sugar, maple syrup)
> ½ teaspoon (2.5 ml) vanilla extract (optional)
> For fixins: ground cinnamon (optional)

1. Mix all powders except cinnamon in a mug.

2. Pour in ½ cup (120 ml) hot water and mix with a fork until powders are all dissolved.

3. Pour in frothed hemp mylk and gently mix.

4. Sweeten to taste and enjoy with an optional dash of cinnamon on top.

Superfood Salt Sprinkle

I love to salt my food rather generously and am grateful for high-quality salts such as Himalayan pink salt and Celtic sea salt, which are rich in essential minerals and nutrients. This recipe enhances the medicine of salt with mineral- and vitamin-rich superfoods, nutritional yeast high in B vitamins, and seeds that support heart health—and give an extra crunch. Sprinkle this on top of salads, roasted veggies, avocados, toast, or a baked sweet potato for added flavor, texture, and nutrition.

Yield: approximately ¼ cup (37 g)

> 1 teaspoon (2.5 g) moringa powder
> 1 teaspoon (4 g) nutritional yeast powder
> 1 teaspoon (2.5 g) black sesame seeds
> 1 teaspoon (2.5 g) hemp seeds
> 8 teaspoons (20 g) Himalayan pink salt or Celtic sea salt
> 1 teaspoon (2.5 g) smoked paprika powder
> 1 teaspoon (2.5 g) black pepper (optional)

1. Mix and store in a small jar. Use often.

Plant Mylks & Marvelous Herbal Mylk Variations

Alternative "mylks" are nutritious, dairy free, easily digestible additions to elixirs, teas, and smoothies and can also be enjoyed on their own either cold or hot. Although long popular with vegans, they have become more popular with nonvegans who wish to avoid cow's milk for health or environmental purposes. I occasionally enjoy a glass of raw milk from a happy, grass-fed cow if I have the privilege of connecting to a farm with lactating dairy cows, but since leaving Vermont, this has become rare, so I make plant mylks as a treat.

Hemp, almond, soy, oat, pea, cashew, and other mylks are readily available at the grocery store, but making one at home is an easy, preservative-free, less expensive way to add nutrition and creaminess to elixirs or teas.

When making mylk, I consider the environmental impact and the nutritional benefits of each plant as well as the texture and taste. My favorites are hemp and oat mylks; almond is delicious, but they are grown in drought-stricken areas of California and have a high water footprint. I try to avoid soy for health and hormonal reasons as well as environmental and political reasons.

Hemp is incredibly nutritious. It's full of protein, minerals, healthy fats, and unsaturated essential fatty acids, which are essential for building new tissue and membranes in your body—in other words, regeneration. The flavor is smooth, it makes a creamy milk, and unlike some other milk alternatives, it even froths well for a cappuccino or elixir! Working with hemp is my preference from an environmental perspective as well, as it is a largely regenerative crop that I hope will be used once again for paper, fiber, medicine, and food. It is a hardy crop that helps build soil and uses less water than almond and cow milks.

However, in terms of water use, oat mylk is the winner. It is not quite as nutritionally dense as hemp, nor does it have as much protein, but it is more nutritious than almond mylk and is smooth and delicious.

Store-bought organic alternative milks can be pricey, but making them at home is inexpensive, easy, quick, and preservative free. They require only water and blending, and you can freeze and save the strained pulp to add to baked goods or oatmeal—no waste! The best part is that making them at home gives you the pleasure of getting creative with inventing herbal alternatives to the simple nut mylks.

Linden Rose Hemp Mylk

Here's a delightful herbal mylk! For a plain hemp or oat mylk, use water as a base.

Yield: About 4 cups (960 ml)

½ cup (3.5 g) hemp seeds

4 cups (960 ml) linden leaf and flower infusion (see page 55); use less water for thicker, creamier milk

1 pinch Himalayan pink sea salt

1 whole date, pitted, or 1 tablespoon maple syrup (20 g) or coconut sugar (9 g) (optional)

½ teaspoon (2.5 ml) vanilla extract (optional)

1 tablespoon (15 ml) Flora Sagrada Rose Hydrosol (optional)

Other delightful possible additions:

2 tablespoons (10 g) cocoa or cacao powder for "Chocolate Lover's Heart Mylk"

¼ cup (38 g) fresh strawberries for "Linden Rose Pink Mylk"

1. Place hemp seeds, herbal infusion (or water for plain mylk), salt, and any add-ins in a blender. Blend on high for about 1 minute or until the mixture seems well combined.

2. Dip in, kitchen witch, and see whether you'd like to add more sweetness, rose, or other flavors.

3. Pour the mixture directly into a serving container or mason jar. You can use a nut-mylk bag to strain it for optimal creamy-smooth mylk, though it is not necessary if you have a high-speed blender.

4. Cover and refrigerate. The mylk will keep in the refrigerator up to 5 days.

Cool Spring Breakfast: Superfood Porridge

This is a great breakfast for anytime between the Fall and early Spring, when we wake up to a crisp, cold morning. It is also great for people who tend to be frail and thin, as it nourishes and grounds a scattered air element and nervous energy. When our digestive fire is still weak and just waking up, a warming, adaptogenic porridge can be something that's easy to digest. Use this recipe as a base or inspiration and allow making the porridge to be a fun and creative process. Listen to what dried fruits, herbs, or mylks your body is craving!

The dried fruit and banana in this version sweeten the porridge without the need for additional sweetener. It is rich in fiber, vitamins, minerals, adaptogens, and healthy fats. You can add a tablespoon (16 g) of almond butter on top or mix in some ghee if you are frail, have air in chaos, or tend toward anxiety and need more grounding.

Yield: 1–2 servings

½ cup (45 g) powdered oats (you can use the blender to make oats into powder yourself)

3 tablespoons (75 g) dried goji berries

2 tablespoons (50 g) chopped dried apples, prunes, cherries, or other fruit

1 tablespoon (9 g) maca powder

1 tablespoon (9 g) mesquite powder

1 teaspoon (4 g) ground cinnamon

½ cup (120 ml) hemp or almond mylk or 1 tablespoon (16 g) almond butter

½ teaspoon (2 g) nutmeg

1 banana

1 tablespoon (10 g) tocos powder (optional)

1 teaspoon (2 g) powdered flaxseed (optional)

3 drops liquid stevia (optional)

1. Combine the powdered oats and 1 cup (240 ml) of spring water in a large pot. Add the dried fruit, maca, mesquite, and cinnamon.

2. Stir and bring to a simmer over low heat until it thickens into a porridge.

3. Stir in the hemp mylk, thinning it. Stir in tocos powder, flaxseed (if using), and stevia (if using).

4. To serve, mash half of the banana into the porridge and slice the other half, serving it on top. Sprinkle the nutmeg on top.

Green Wild Egg Scramble

This is my favorite springtime recipe, and I make it each year when I take students camping. Part of the process is seeing which wild weeds are abundant; when I take the Gaia School apprentices, we each forage a handful, and I create a large scramble for everyone. Children have been converted into green-eating foragers by this dish and have delighted their parents by eagerly starting to forage weeds at home for breakfast!

Yield: 4 servings

4 handfuls abundant weed of your choice (young mallow leaves and nettles are my favorites!)

6 farm-fresh organic eggs

1–2 tablespoons (15–30 ml) grass-fed butter or olive oil

Celtic salt and black pepper to taste

Smoked chipotle pepper to taste (optional)

3 tablespoons (28 g) goat cheese (optional)

1. Roughly chop the weeds and place them onto a large preheated pan over medium heat. Add ½ cup (120 ml) water and quickly cover, letting the weeds steam.

2. Uncover after a few seconds to check. When the herbs are steamed and the water is gone, use a spatula to make a hole in the center of the weeds.

3. Turn heat to low, put a generous amount of butter in the hole to melt, and break the eggs into the melted butter.

4. Sprinkle Celtic sea salt over the eggs and allow the whites to slowly cook.

5. When the whites look half done, add goat cheese, if using, in large chunks onto the eggs.

6. Gently break the egg yolks with the spatula, stirring the yolks, melting the cheese into the whites, and, finally, stirring everything into the greens.

7. Serve with fresh ground pepper and smoked chipotle sauce or powder for a little extra kick.

Wild Greens Salad with Edible Flowers

Spring is the time of fresh, wild greens. In some parts of the world, we can walk through forests and meadows eating and feasting on abundant wild food. Get to know your local edible wild weeds and enjoy developing relationships to the wilderness around your home all year round so you can enjoy giving to the land and receiving from her too.

Some wild weeds that make a delicious green base:

- Chickweed (sweet and delicate)
- Miner's lettuce (sweet and delicate)
- Wild strawberry leaf
- Violet leaf and flower
- Young dandelion greens (slightly bitter; use sparingly)
- Young mallow leaves (a little hairy and thicker; use sparingly)
- Young plantain leaves
- Young wild mustard (tastes like wasabi; use as a spicy accent)
- Young yarrow leaves (a little bitter and not juicy; use sparingly)
- Wood sorrel leaf and flower (delicate and delicious lemon flavor; use sparingly)
- Nasturtium leaves
- Wild radish leaves and young seed pods (delicious, juicy, and spicy)

Edible flowers to sprinkle onto your salad:

- Red clover (best to pull apart and sprinkle)
- Wild radish
- Wild or garden arugula (spicy and delicious)
- Mustard flower (spicy and delicious)
- Dandelion flower (pull apart and sprinkle)
- Elderflower (stay away from toxic leaves and stems)
- Evening primrose
- Rose (pull apart and sprinkle petals)
- Calendula flower (pull apart and sprinkle petals)
- Borage flowers
- Nasturtium flowers (spicy, juicy, and delicious)
- Rosemary flowers

My secret to a delicious salad is getting all of the flavors (sweet, salty, pungent, bitter, and sour) and a variety of textures (crispy, soft, and juicy) in a single bowl.

My go-to salad uses greens as a base, edible flowers from the garden, and the following additions: I slice a juicy, crisp apple (such as a Honeycrisp, Fuji, or Granny Smith) in cubes, add either dried cherries or dried cranberries, and toast pumpkin seeds, sunflower seeds, or pecans in a pan on the stove. I often add avocados, drizzle with lemon juice and olive oil, and sprinkle with a good salt. This salad is so hydrating, satisfying, and delicious, even children love it. When I have picky eaters, I'll drizzle a little maple syrup into the dressing, and all the greens get eaten.

Herbal-Infused Apple Cider Vinegar

Herbal vinegars are a staple in the herbalist's apothecary and are something the kitchen Witch can use daily. Raw, fermented apple cider vinegar is already food medicine—it is great for digestion and full of enzymes; it lowers blood sugar levels and boosts immunity. As a medicine-making Green Witch, this is my favorite menstruum for extracting the medicinal properties of nourishing herbs. While making an alcohol tincture (see pages 120 to 122) of nettles or chickweed feels too strong for me, making a vinegar of the wild weeds becomes a harmonious form of herbal food medicine. Apple cider vinegar beautifully extracts minerals and vitamins from our nourishing plants. Adding aromatic, mineral-rich herbs such as lemon balm, lemon verbena, tulsi, and mint adds wonderful flavor and enhances the digestive support of the apple cider vinegar.

You can use your herbal vinegar in cooking—add it to rice, stir-fries, salad dressings, and soups. To strengthen your digestive system and ward off colds, you can also begin the practice of drinking a glass of water with 1 to 2 tablespoons (15 to 30 ml) of your herbal vinegar each morning on an empty stomach. And sipping on 1 tablespoon (15 ml) of your vinegar in ½ cup (120 ml) of water during or after a meal has been shown to lower blood-sugar levels.

Here are some variations. Get creative! Have fun inventing your own blends in the Spring and stock your apothecary for the year when weeds are abundant.

Nettle–Lemon Balm Vinegar

Yield: varies

> Fresh, roughly chopped nettles or other nourishing herb
> Roughly chopped fresh lemon balm, lemon verbena, mint, holy basil, or basil
> Raw apple cider vinegar

1. Use any size jar. Fill it half full of fresh, roughly chopped nettles or another nourishing herb of your choice.

2. Fill the other half with roughly chopped fresh lemon balm, lemon verbena, mint, holy basil, or basil. Leave about an inch at the top of your jar so the herbs do not stick out of your menstruum.

3. Pour organic, raw apple cider vinegar over the herbs and push them down with a wooden spoon so the herbs are completely submerged. Cover with wax paper, as vinegar can react with a jar lid, and seal your jar.

4. Shake, label, and store in a dark place, shaking every few days and whispering encouragement and love to the infusing herbs.

5. After 4 to 8 weeks, strain, bottle, and keep in your fridge. Use as often as possible.

Help-Me-Digest Vinegar

Herbal bitters promote the production of bile and digestive enzymes. So does apple cider vinegar. Thus, my favorite menstruum for herbal bitters is apple cider vinegar instead of a traditional alcohol-based tincture. Again, get creative and witchy—have fun in this Spring portal of expansive play and alchemy! Here is a simple herbal bitter using mugwort. Mugwort is very bitter in flavor and is an ally for folks with irritable bowel syndrome or acid reflux. A bitter is working physiologically in the body when you taste the flavor in your mouth, so do not sweeten your herbal bitters. Instead, just take a few small sips diluted in water 20 minutes before a meal to prepare your digestive system; you can also take small sips during your meal. When struggling with digestion, do not drink cold beverages during a meal as they will dilute the digestive juices we are stimulating with the herbal bitters.

Yield: varies

> Dried mugwort or fresh leaves
> Raw apple cider vinegar

1. Fill a jar one-third full with dried mugwort or three-quarters full with fresh leaves.

2. Pour the raw apple cider vinegar into the jar to top it off.

3. Allow it to infuse in a dark cabinet and strain after 4 to 8 weeks. Keep it in your fridge.

Herbal-Infused White Vinegar for Spring Cleaning

As a Green Witch, I call upon my plant allies in all aspects of my life, including the cleansing and activating of my home space. One day, as I was harvesting lavender blossoms for tea, the spirit of the lavender told me to harvest the leaves and stems as well and infuse them in white vinegar for cleaning. Indeed, this part of the plant is often left unused, but it holds the medicinal and aromatic essential oils of lavender. Thus, this beautiful recipe was born, guided by my plants and garden. Washing your surfaces with this herbal cleaning solution feels like anointing a temple with the songs of the plants and the Spring gusts of wind!

Yield: varies

> Aromatic plant, such as lavender, rosemary, eucalyptus, pine, or mint
> White vinegar

1. Roughly chop your plant. Fill a jar or other sealable container to about 80 percent full.

2. Pour the vinegar into jar to top it off. Close tightly.

3. Let vinegar infuse for a couple of months in a dark cupboard.

4. Strain. Dilute 2 parts vinegar with 1 part water. Optional: Add 1 tablespoon (15 ml) Castile soap, such as Dr. Bronners, and/or add 5 to 13 drops of lavender or eucalyptus essential oil. Test your spray to see if you wish to adjust the aroma.

5. Use to clean your home and bring in the aromatic brightness and cleansing properties of the healing herbs.

Raw Herbal Juices

Making a raw herbal juice is a wonderful skill taught to me by Sage Maurer. It comes from folk herbalists in tropical countries, where it is not as common to dry plants for medicine. Medicinal plants grow all year near the equator, and the humidity makes it hard to dry herbs, so herbalists do not rely on dried ingredients as much as they do in the European folk-medicine traditions I come from. I am so grateful to Sage for teaching me this method of making fresh medicine, as it has become one of my favorite ways to work with the herbs in the Spring, when nourishing wild weeds are abundant and delicious to enjoy fresh.

To make an herbal juice such as the following two, simply add a handful of fresh herbs into a blender full of water, blend, and strain! Blending stinging nettles into a pesto or juice eliminates the sting without needing to heat the herb; do strain the juice, however. Blending a gentle herb, such as chickweed in a high-speed blender often does not require straining. Get creative with the weeds that grow around you! See the Summer chapter for more herbal juice recipes.

Spring Cleanse Herbal Juice

Yield: 2 to 4 servings

> 2 handfuls fresh chickweed (or other weed)
> ½ handful fresh lemon verbena leaves or a handful of fresh lemon balm leaves (optional)
> 4-inch (10 cm) section of inner aloe pulp or 4 tablespoons (60 ml) fresh aloe juice (optional)

1. Add ingredients to a blender full of spring water.

2. Blend on high, strain, and serve over ice or bottle and store in the refrigerator.

Nettle-Mint Juice

Yield: 2 to 4 servings

> 2 handfuls fresh nettles
> 2 handfuls fresh mint (optional)
> Blender full of spring water, or use strong chilled mint tea if not using fresh mint

1. Blend, strain, and enjoy cold.

· · · · · · · ·

Mother Earth's Breast Milk

This fresh juice recipe is a miraculous gift from the wild Earth available for about a two-week window each spring, when the wild green oats mature into their milky oat tops. When the tops can be squeezed and release a drop of white milk, the nourishing *Avena sativa* becomes even more powerfully restorative to the nervous system.

Yield: 2 to 4 servings

> 3 large handfuls of milky oat tops (page 95)
> Water

1. Collect the milky oat tops following the sacred harvesting guidelines on pages 34 to 35 and put three large handfuls into a blender full of water.

2. Blend and strain.

You will get a creamy, light green elixir that tastes like a fresh, lightly grassy, creamy Spring milk. Your body will instantly feel relaxed, calm, and deeply nourished. Upon drinking this elixir that feels like Gaia's breastmilk, you will feel your heart opening and softening as a surge of vitality and energy moves through your body. Read more about the medicinal properties of *Avena sativa* in the plant profiles of Spring.

FLOWER ESSENCES

In the Spring, flowers sing. Making flower essences is a magickal way Green Witches bring healing—by flooding the energetic frequencies of our bodies and souls with the vibrations and sacred geometry of flowers. Like homeopathy, flower essences heal through vibrations. They are diluted and should be taken often. Making a flower essence is a magickal ritual between a Witch, the flower spirit that speaks to her soul, and the elements of fire (sun), water, earth (flower), and air (pollen). Legends say that the ancient medicine people of Lemuria and Atlantis used flower essences to heal. I have received secret instructions on how to receive flower essences made by Nature and have seen the profound and magickal shifts the purity of the flowers awaken in humans. Dr. Edward Bach, who made flower essences famous in the West, deserted orthodox medicine upon seeing how simple and effective the vibrational healing of the flowers is. It is said that in the presence of the vibration of the flowers, dis-ease melts away like snow.

To make a flower essence, you will need a pure and open heart, a clean crystal vessel or clear jar half full of spring water, your journal, and an offering for the plants.

Prepare yourself by cleansing your body and spirit physically with sacred smoke or prayer. You may only harvest plants with an open heart full of gratitude and a peaceful spirit. Pray, call in the directions, meditate with a tea, do the Earth body harmonizing ritual on page 91—do what you need to do to harmonize your energy.

Cast forth your prayer, asking a flower to choose you. Even if you love a particular flower and imagine wanting to make an essence of it, stay open to the alchemy between you and any flower in the moment of this ritual. Your vibration and the vibration of a flower will match to allow for the transformation needed in your frequency at this time. The flower that is singing to your heart now may surprise you; as you walk through your garden or wild land with an open heart, listen for the one your heart connects to.

Once you find the flower, sit down with her and introduce yourself. Make an offering and explain why you are here. Spend some time together so your energy can connect, and give her your full attention and presence. Observe her from the perspective of a bug. With your head on the soil looking up, follow the veins in her petals. Pretend you are a bee. What do you see? What do you feel? Open your heart and notice what she is sharing with you. You may choose to meditate with her, exchange energy through your open palms, or continue falling deeper into her with your loving gaze and listening heart. The flowers have guided me to work with affirmations when being graced by their energy. So I ask for the flower to share an affirmation with me about her vibration, her song. Write what comes through in your journal.

Once you feel a clear transmission of what she has shared with you, you will already feel the shift of energy inside of you and the healing of her song in your heart. Now you may ask permission to harvest the flower. If you feel a yes, place your open jar half full of spring water under the plant and pinch the flower so she falls

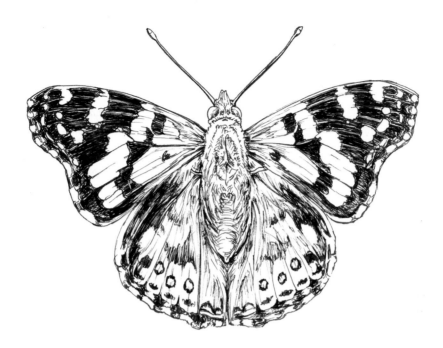

onto the surface of the water, ideally facing up. Set the jar at the base of her mother plant, on the Earth, in the direct sunlight. The light of the sun will transfer the sacred geometric life-force vibration of the flower into the receptive body of the water over a period of roughly three hours. After three hours have passed, remove the flower with a stem or your fingers without touching the water, and top off the flower essence with brandy. This is your Mother Essence—it is now a jar half full of pure essence and half full of brandy. Shake this jar, speaking the affirmation into the essence through your heart and giving gratitude. Label the jar with the name of the flower, the affirmation, and the date and location. Give gratitude and offerings to the plant.

You may now make a stock essence, which you may generously share with your friends, spreading the healing song of the flower to the human race. Fill a small jar or dropper bottle (4 oz, 120 ml, will do) with an equal amount of brandy and water. Drop seven drops of the Mother Stock into this mixture and shake while speaking the affirmation and beaming it from your heart. Often, folks are taught to make a third

dilution, a dosage bottle, by filling another glass jar with a brandy/water mixture and adding a few drops of the stock to the dosage bottle. However, I prefer to work with the stock essence, adding it to my waters, teas, and so on.

When working with a flower essence, make a few stock bottles and place one near your bathtub, one near your source of drinking water, one in your purse, one in your car, one by your bed, and the like. With flower essences, we tune ourselves frequently to the song of the plants until our bodies can hold that vibration. Then we "graduate" to a different flower essence. To use it, add a few drops to your water bottle, bathtub, facial mist, food, and so on. Use it often. When drinking it in or dropping it under your tongue, speak your affirmation and know in your heart, soul, and all of your singing cells that it is done! And so it is!

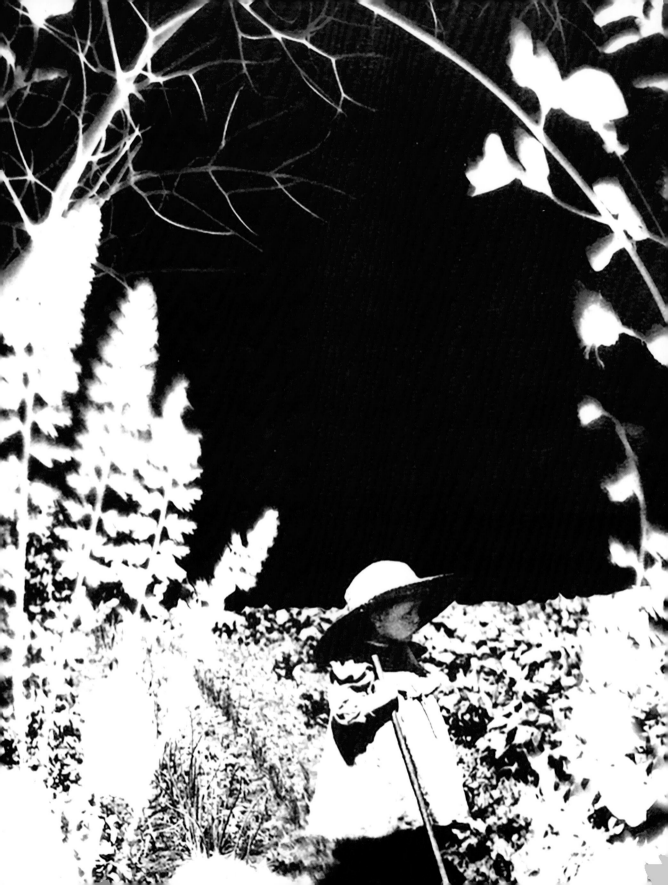

In the Garden, on the Earth

Spring is the time to plant both metaphorical and literal seeds so we can enjoy a fruitful and abundant summer.

In the Spring, we delight in, dream of, and plan the garden we will be cultivating all Summer. Begin by noticing what you already have. What plants naturally grow around your home? Maybe a previous landowner planted bulbs that come up each Spring. How can you enhance the existing perennial expression of the season?

As tenders of the Earth, we seek to encourage and support growth and beauty without making changes to the landscape that are too harsh or deep. How can you support what you already have and expand on it? What areas around your home have good soil? Where will seeds easily take? Spend time observing your land and garden throughout all the seasons to make the best choices come Spring. Start small. Each Spring you can add layers of transformation, learning what takes and what dreams and visions did not come into fruition. In permaculture, we observe land for a full year before implementing any changes. This prevents us from putting a lot of energy (time, money, plants, soil) into an action that may not be of greatest benefit to the ecosystem. We seek to build on the energy that is present, alchemizing our efforts with Nature, so the whole can be greater than the sum of its parts— allowing both the land and our human communities to thrive.

In the wild, we may visit areas we tend and harvest from, greeting the rebirth of the plants with whom we are in relationship. In the early Spring, I often venture out to my secret harvest spots just to visit and say hello, as if greeting a newborn. It feels wonderful to see my beloved plant friends waking up from their Winter slumber, and I leave prayers and offerings. As they mature, I go and harvest wild weeds that are growing in abundance to dry or make herbal vinegars (see pages 79 to 80). Spring is also a wonderful time to learn plant IDs and to observe how plants change as they grow and mature. Some young weeds, such as thistle and mustard, are delightful to eat when they are just babies, and as they grow, they change and become less of a treat in flavor and texture.

Permaculture and Regenerative Farming Practices

Ideally, observe the land you steward for at least a year, noticing how water flows and where it pools in the rainy seasons, and how the sun moves. What parts of your garden have sunlight in the Winter months, when the trees drop leaves but the sun is low? Where does the sun hit in the Summer? Where is that perfect place of balance with ample light and moist, rich soil? Consider your climate. If you live in the northern United States, for example, it is ideal to plant your Summer garden where it will be fully revealed to the sun, because the growing season is short and frequent summer rainstorms will keep the garden moist. In areas such as Southern California, where the summers are hot and dry, however, your garden may thrive with some protection from nearby trees or shrubs. In these Mediterranean climates, deciduous trees will drop their leaves in the winter when your garden needs all the sun it can get. These trees will also create moisture and shade in the oppressive Summer heat so your vegetables don't burn.

Consider how you move through the land you tend, planning your food garden closest to your kitchen and home. In permaculture, we plan zones based on areas we frequently use and the space they require. While a kitchen garden does not need to be large to produce a lot of food, an orchard, for example, requires more space. It also requires fewer daily visits, so it can be planted further away from the home.

Find the places that are ready to become gardens for food, perennial herbs, or flowers and notice where the soil is struggling. In those places, focus on building soil. This is an important prerequisite for a thriving garden. Each time you grow plants, you should also grow soil. Planting cover crops is a terrific way to heal the Earth and build topsoil.

Regenerative farmers heal depleted land by changing the way it is being farmed. You can do this on a smaller scale. If you are starting with rock-hard, compacted soil, learn the no-till method of regenerative farming. Rather than tilling land, which releases carbon into the air and kills the life of soil, plant daikon radishes the

first year. Their roots penetrate hard soil, and when they decompose, they add nitrogen, nutrients, and biology. Plant a mixture of cover crops—nitrogen-fixing plants such as sweet peas and vetch. When they are green and just starting to flower, "chop and drop": cut them, water them, cover them with hay or alfalfa, and create a layer of composting mulch on the soil. Within one season of planting cover crops in poor soil, you may be able to effortlessly glide your hand into rich, lively black soil that will make your garden thrive, where seeds will easily take, and that will grow nutrient-rich food. After all, vegetables and fruit are only as nutritious as the soil in which they grow! Furthermore, building soil and employing regenerative farming practices feeds your small water cycle, replenishing groundwater, sequestering carbon from the atmosphere, and helping to reverse the climate change crisis. It is empowering and uplifting to realize how much positive change we can create for our planet in our very own backyard! Don't let it intimidate you—start by planting a cover crop mix. The garden will teach you; the soil speaks too.

Pollinators, Perennials, Life, and Death

When planting a garden, ensure you are supporting an ecosystem of pollinators. Mixing in native wildflowers and perennial herbs that attract hummingbirds, bees, and butterflies will help you and your garden thrive. Planting a diverse range of plants is beneficial. Visually, you can plant clusters together while ensuring diversity over the whole space. It is best to release the expectation of a manicured garden. Whatever you do, do not take leaf litter and plant material off your property—rather, scatter it at the base of the plants to build mulch. If you can't bear the sight of it, use a mulch you find visually appealing or plant a groundcover so the soil is never exposed and compost the leaf litter onsite. Consider adding a bird bath to enjoy the presence of birds. Invite life in! Diversity encourages a thriving environment. Invite death in! A garden rich in decay and compost is the garden where life effortlessly grows.

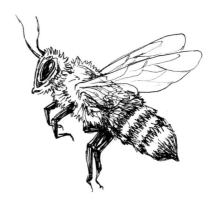

GUERRILLA GARDENING

If you live in an urban environment or frequent areas that have empty lots, sidewalk strips, or any other parcels of land that are not being loved, consider secretly adopting a patch of public space. Find out what native seeds grow best in your area and scatter them at night with prayers to rewild our cities! Get together with your friends and make seed bombs—little balls of seeds, compost, clay, and sand—that you can throw into empty spaces to disintegrate with the rain, releasing seeds and compost. I have been known to drive by urban lots and throw seed bombs out of my car window. How much fun can you have being radical in your love of a healthy ecosystem? How generous can you be in planting seeds for people and places other than yourself? The pollinators that are looking for food in urban places will find the little plant sanctuaries you create for them. A wildflower will tickle the heart of a child. Beauty and play can heal us too.

WHAT TO DO IN THE SPRING

Garden Tasks

- Plant seeds!

- Start seeds indoors to transplant into the garden (tomatoes, squash, basil, and other summer annuals).

- Plant wildflowers directly in the ground.

- Turn your compost pile.

- Plant living mulch (a spring blend of cover crops).

- Let weeds grow. If you must, chop them at the base, leaving the root in the ground so it does not disturb the important living network in the soil.

- Plan your garden.

- Go to your local nursery.

- Plant bulbs and perennial herbs and flowers.

- Plant fruit trees.

- Feed your garden with compost and/or compost tea.

Apothecary Tasks

- Harvest wild weeds and dry them to have the nourishment of spring all year around. You can do this with nettles, chickweed, raspberry leaf, and cleavers, for example.

- Make nourishing herbal vinegars, extracting the mineral and nutrient-rich properties of the wild weeds in apple cider vinegar.

- Make herbal bitters for digestion.

- Make flower essences.

- Craft glyercerines of flowers and fresh young herbs.

- Eat wild food and edible flowers.

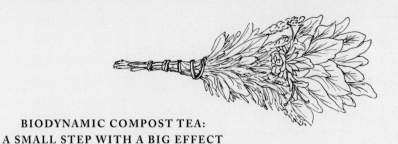

BIODYNAMIC COMPOST TEA:
A SMALL STEP WITH A BIG EFFECT

Rudolf Steiner, the grandfather of biodynamic agriculture, was a brilliant visionary, inventor, and awakened human. His practice of making biodynamic compost is an accessible practice that is remarkably healing to land and plants, growing the highest caliber of food with the greatest nutritional profiles.

Biodynamic practices can get complicated, but this is an easy practice you can do on your own if you can get your hands on some biodynamic compost, which is becoming more readily available. For more information on biodynamic agriculture—and to purchase biodynamic preps—visit the Josephine Porter Institute online (jpibiodynamics.org).

> You will need:
>
> - A 5-gallon (19 L) bucket
> - 2 handfuls of biodynamic compost
> - Water
> - A branch with leaves, a hand broom, or a toilet brush for this use only (as taught by my dear teacher farmer Jack)

Place the compost in the bucket and add water until the bucket is about 80 percent full. Using a straight arm, swirl the mixture, creating a vortex like a tornado. Then swish it in the opposite direction. Steiner said these two spiraling movements represent and bring in the energies of universal order and universal chaos, from which all of the Great Web is made. Let your intentions for the health of your land and the Earth pour from your heart, through your hand into the receptive body of water and compost tea. Do this for a few minutes. When it begins to feel silkier, it is activated and ready.

Dip your branch or brush into the bucket and bless the plants and land with this gentle atmospheric and foliar spray; draw your hand back behind your body and move it forward as if you were throwing a ball, letting the drops of tea fall onto the earth. You do not need much, and it is beneficial to coat the leaves, which absorb the nutrients from the spray.

You can refer to a biodynamic calendar (there are free versions online) to see whether it is a leaf day, flower day, fruit day, or root day. Depending on the energetics of the day, your application will feed the energies of that aspect of the plant's production. For instance, if you want to encourage your roses to bloom, spray on a flower day. If your roses have rusty leaves, spray on a leaf day. If a plant is struggling, repeat daily or every other day several times until you see improvement.

Spring Rituals

As humans, we rely on the rebirth of nature. The rituals that weave us into the awakening of life and land are some of the most ancient practices of our ancestors that we continue today. Easter and Passover, for example, draw on ancient pagan rituals that celebrate and attune us to the rebirth of Spring. Easter celebrates the resurrection of the "sun God," Christ. It weaves in the delight of children finding eggs in a garden, young lamb roasted on the fire, and rituals of cleansing and blessing water. The symbols predate the Christian holiday. The rabbit is an ancient symbol of the Goddess; the egg is a symbol of the universe. Druids are said to have painted eggs red like menstrual blood and buried them in freshly plowed fields to feed the fertility of the Earth.

The rituals of Passover take us from the emotional misery of death and darkness associated with the archetype of the long winter dark night, to the joyful, long-awaited rebirth of a people with a new life on new land. The various sacred food rituals associated with the Passover meal include bitter spring greens and invite in the participation of children—weaving in the energies of youth, vitality, and innocence.

Following are some of my most important Spring rituals. Many of them are very simple and have profound effects in shifting and renewing our energy.

Flower Mandalas and Courting the Earth

As we move on the Great Wheel through the energies of Spring and the maturing Maiden, we enter portals of fertility, ecstasy, and courting the beloved. Rituals of devotion and offerings to the Earth are a wonderful way to weave the energies of Spring into the Great Romance that is taking place all around you. How can you be the most devoted lover to the Earth? What does it mean to be in loving relationship with Nature? How do you court the Beloved? What does it feel like to sing songs to the dawn, leave flowers for the fairies, and create random acts of beauty and kindness?

Creating a flower mandala in the spring is such a practice. As the poet Rumi said, "Let the beauty we love be what we do. There are hundreds of ways to kneel and kiss the ground."

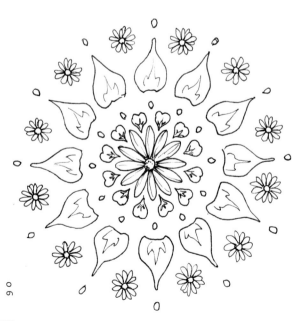

Allow the ritual to be in the gathering of the flowers. Walk through your garden with a prayer, asking which flowers wish to become an offering of beauty. Harvest them with gratitude and collect them into your basket. Alternatively, create a flower mandala in your community, inviting everyone to bring flowers. Set the intention for the mandala and invite this ritual to occur without verbal communication, but rather with the intention of working together like a hive of bees, in harmony and alchemy. Invite your friends to leave the flowers on the Earth and begin intuitively arranging them. Before beginning, when setting the intention of working like a hive, I share that it is okay to move other people's flowers without attachment to our part of the creation—that the whole is greater than the sum of its parts. And so we create beauty and finally step back to take it in. End by holding hands, sometimes speaking prayers or a dedication of the offering to the Earth.

Earth My Body: Harmonizing Your Body with the Earth Mother's Body

The Earth's magnetic field vibrates at 7.83 Hertz, which is called the Schumann Resonance. Scientists are now finding evidence that "earthing," or connecting our bare feet or bodies to the surface of the Earth for twenty minutes a day, has a profound healing and anti-inflammatory effect on the body. Astronauts who travel into space have a machine that creates this electromagnetic vibration. We are like plants—unrooted and disconnected from the Earth, we become isolated, get ill, and die.

You can harmonize your body with the Earth daily for optimal health and well-being. Although it weaves us into the Earth energy of the North portal, it is often when Gaia begins awakening in the Spring that this practice becomes available. It feels deeply grounding and calming, but it is surprisingly energizing as well. Upon coming into harmony, you should feel at peace in your mind, relaxed in your body, uplifted in your heart, and renewed in spirit.

1. Walk into Nature—your garden, a park, or anywhere you can access the body of the Earth.

2. Lie down. I recommend you start on your back. Close your eyes, lay your palms on the Earth or your belly and heart, and begin to breathe deeply, releasing tension each time you exhale.

3. Spend a few minutes feeling your mind settle and your body relax. Feel the support of the Earth holding you. Often five minutes is all it takes to feel a profound difference in your energy and a grounding.

4. Then flip over. You will find a whole new layer is available when you lay your body the other way against the belly of the Mother. Again, close your eyes, breathe, relax, let go, and receive from the Earth.

This is my favorite practice to do before any ceremony, teaching, or ritual. It is the quickest and most profound way to come into harmony with the Earth's healing vibration, and all it takes is ten to twenty minutes. Of course, you can do this for hours, which feels utterly divine. The longer you lay your body on the Earth, the more portals open.

Egg Cleansing

This ritual, a form of limpia ceremony, was shared with me by a shamanic teacher as well as women in Mexico. It is a folk practice found in many cultures, though I have predominantly found it woven into Latin American folk remedies. I humbly pass it on with permission, though I am of Polish descent. Many of my Latina Gaia Witches have laughed when I share it, saying that their mothers and aunties do this—and if one of them has a headache or is stressed, they will call out, "Get the huevo!" My heart has had the blessing of witnessing my sisters of Latina heritage weep in the reclamation of this beautiful ceremony—it is so simple, yet so profound and healing. What we sometimes reject as Maidens returns to us on the spiral dance, and it may become a practice that weaves us with our ancestors.

This ceremony cleanses the energetic body of negative and dense energies. It is also used to relieve energy that causes stress and tension headaches. It is very calming and purifying to the heart. You can do it in the home, though I prefer to do it outside and to do it for someone and receive from someone, rather than doing it for myself.

My young daughter and I will often do this together, laying a blanket in the garden and offering each other an egg cleansing or full-body massage with the egg. Flora likes it when I have one egg in each hand and work on her body with both as she lies on the Earth with her eyes closed. The result is always a purified spirit and gentle, open heart full of wonder and awe.

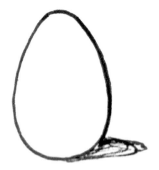

You will need:
An egg, preferably one from a chicken that has had a happy, natural life

1. Holding the egg in your hand, close your eyes. Connect to your prayer or intention.

2. Rub the egg all over your or the other person's body. Start with the head, massage the face and neck, and move all the way down to the toes.

3. Notice how the egg pulls dense energy from the body, making you or the person you're working on feel lighter.

4. Return the egg to the Earth, giving gratitude.

Sacred Seed Planting

Any time you plant seeds, you have the opportunity to weave your intentions, prayers, and even biological needs into the miracle of the seed and its potential.

You will need:
Seeds

1. Observe the seeds you hold with the eyes of a child. Be in wonder and awe! Each seed is different in size, texture, shape, and color—study them as a world.

2. Open your heart to the feeling of eternity held in the moment of this seed and of your seed spell. This seed comes from ancient lineages, has stories of diverse lands, and holds the prayers and preferences of people who cultivated it, protected it, and spread it over generations, allowing it to arrive to you. It also has the potential of living into eternal futures; just this one seed will become a plant with potentially thousands of seeds, each one of those able to make thousands more.

3. Now allow your prayers and intentions to feel the vastness they are entering! Picture the potential, the avenues of time and timelessness.

4. Pray into the seeds. My preferred method is lying on the Earth (after harmonizing my body with it—see page 91) and laying the seeds on my womb or belly. If they are small, I often cup them in my hands and hold my hands to my heart. You may whisper or speak directly into the seeds.

5. A different method of transferring your energy into the seeds is to place them under your tongue for a minute. Envision your intentions or simply lie on the Earth and allow the darkness of your body and the information of your biology to transfer energetically through your saliva. Then place the seeds onto the palm of your hand and hold them to the sun, speaking your prayers, casting a spell with balanced lunar and solar energies.

6. Plant your seeds into the dark flesh of the Earth Mother.

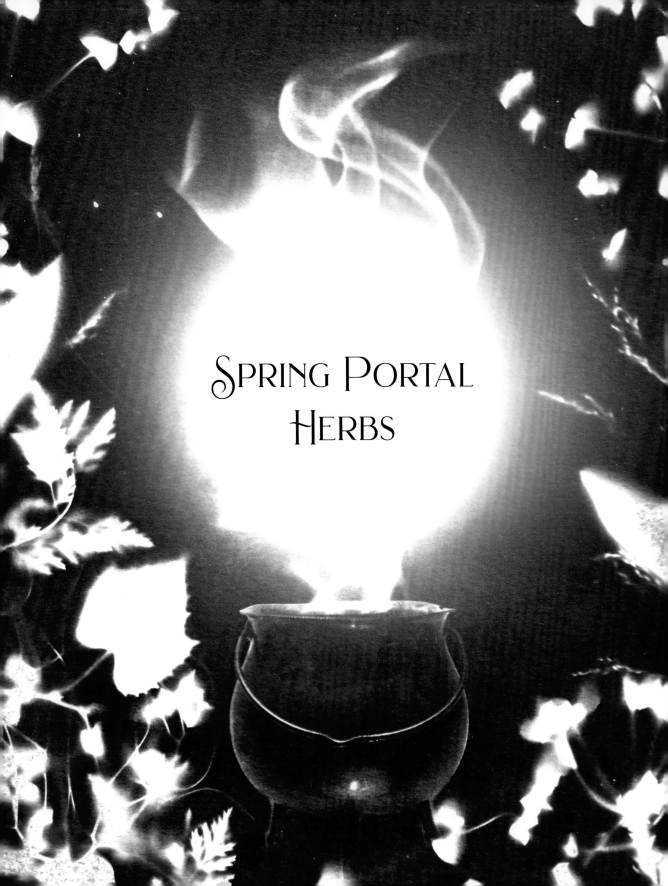

Spring Portal Herbs

plant profile

Oat Straw

LATIN NAME *Avena sativa*

FAMILY Gramineae (grass family)

An annual grass native to northern Europe, now covering meadows and hills worldwide, oat straw grows peacefully and happily in poor, dry soil. Her green fields dance in the spring wind, are cultivated for oatmeal, and turn golden in the late-Summer sun. Each plant grows up to 4 feet (1.2 m) tall, with a hollow jointed stem. The pale green leaves are narrow and flat, and the green flowers are born in loose terminal clusters, with each spikelet consisting of two florets. You can pop the oat tops to release a drop of white "milk" before they turn to grain. The flowers are hermaphroditic and are pollinated by the wind.

HERBAL AND MEDICINAL PROPERTIES

- Nutritive tonic and nourishing herb, both food and medicine: rich in protein, fats, minerals, vitamin B, and fixed oils (source of vitamin E)
- Cardiac tonic: strengthening to the heart and a wonderful ally for lowering cholesterol
- Nervine: calming, relaxing, and restorative to the nervous system; it brings a state of peace and calm while also energizing the body when used consistently
- External emollient: soothing and moistening to inflamed skin; calms eczema, rashes, etc.
- Strengthening ally for times of stress, lifting us out of depression
- Increases stamina and sexual vigor; balances hormones

PLANT SPIRIT HEALING

Oat straw's gently nourishing spirit feels like a sunny breeze and a moist meadow. In times of stress and nervous-system overwhelm, call on the spirit of oat straw to transport you to the peace and bliss of a field with dancing green grasses and grazing horses. There, she will soothe your nerves as you rest and lie on her fertile soil, flooding your body with all the nutrients it needs so it can relax and trust that it is taken care of. Your heart will grow in strength and confidence, and after you have rested and restored, you may feel a surge of energy and joy that calls you to run through the fields like a child. Oat straw brings youth and vitality back to those who have become bitter or closed. She builds trust and balance in the heart, mind, and solar plexus, increasing self-love, confidence, and feelings of inner peace and harmony. Vital, nourished, and connected, we find a renewal of stamina and enthusiasm for life.

FAVORITE USES

- Hot overnight infusion (drink daily for a month or more)
- With other nourishing herbs in tea blends
- Oat-mylk tincture, a favorite nervine
- Fresh milky oat juice (Mother's Earth Breast Milk, page 81)
- Oat seeds with chamomile flowers in the bath for children, to calm and soothe
- Face masks of hydrated oats, rubbed as gentle exfoliant

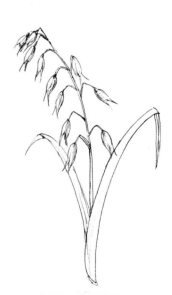

plant profile

Burdock

LATIN NAME *Arctium lappa*

FAMILY Asteraceae/Compositae (aster family)

Native to Europe and Asia, burdock is a common weed growing in temperate regions throughout the world. Often found in meadows, in woods, and at the side of the road, burdock favors disturbed Earth and draws deep nourishment from his long taproot, healing the earth. The root is prized as a detoxifying herb in both Western and Chinese medicine and may be dug up in the fall of the first year of growth. Burdock is a biennial plant with a tall stalk and huge, wavy leaves that grows 6 to 10 feet (1.8 to 3 m) in height and 3 feet (0.9 m) in width. You can recognize it by its pinkish-purple flowers and the brown burrs that stick like Velcro. The taproot is up to 3 feet (0.9 m) long.

HERBAL AND MEDICINAL PROPERTIES

- Nutritive, nourishing herb for restorative food medicine
- Rich in inulins: aids in absorption of nutrients, digestion
- Detoxifying: cleansing to the blood, decongesting to the liver
- Alterative: improves the functioning of the organs of elimination
- Lymphatic: cleansing to the lymphatic system
- Clears skin eruptions, psoriasis, eczema, acne, and irritations associated with body trying to detoxify and being overtaxed
- Diuretic
- Has antimicrobial, antiviral properties
- Anticarcinogenic: supportive for treating cancer
- Nourishes the reproductive system, nervous system, immune system, and digestive system, grounding the body while gently and deeply cleansing old energies, emotions, and toxins

PLANT SPIRIT HEALING

Burdock is a deeply grounding, strengthening, nourishing, and supportive plant spirit that can gently yet effectively go to the root of the wound, moving old, stagnant energy out. The Earthy root is healing and supportive to the root chakra and moves the water element in the body, purifying the emotional realms and nourishing the creative center of the sacral chakra. Consistent use of burdock creates gentle yet deep transformation in the solar plexus and digestive system, strengthening and unclogging the systems and organs of elimination. Often, when we begin working with burdock, our body begins to dig deep and we eliminate more from our bowels, our metabolism comes into greater balance, and we feel emotionally and spiritually lighter as well. Burdock's plant spirit often offers incredible support through a period of healing— allowing our souls to feel held, nourished, and deeply loved. The energy often feels like a safe masculine energy, and I have witnessed a great number of healings occur in which the inner masculine and inner feminine aspect have come into greater harmony within a person, where anger to the masculine washed away and an embodied experience of what a safe masculine energy feels like nourishes and offers healing to an aspect of the body, heart, and soul.

FAVORITE USES

- Overnight hot infusion of dried or fresh herb (drink for a month or more)
- Food medicine: Add to rice, soup stock, bone broth, vegetable purée

OTHER USES

- Leaves can be used for poultices
- Love spells

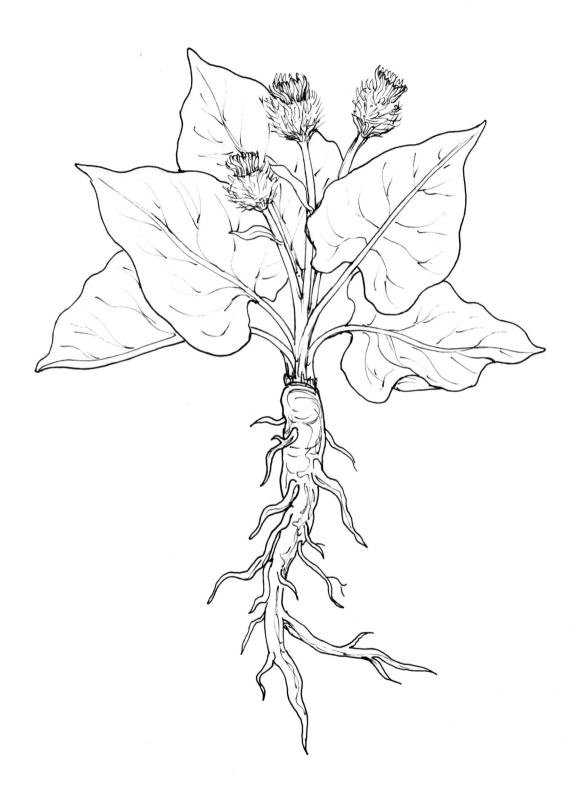

plant profile
Stinging Nettles

LATIN NAME: *Urtica dioica*

FAMILY: Urticaceae (nettle family)

This perennial medicinal weed grows wild worldwide and has been used since ancient times for food, fiber, medicine, and magick. Nettles favor forests, woodlands, and moist soils. They often spread in a large cluster, each plant growing up to 3 to 6 feet (0.9 to 1.8 m) with a width of 2 to 3 feet (0.6 to 0.9 m). Their serrated leaves come to a point and are covered with stinging hairs, as is the stem. In the Spring, the nettle's tender green leaves are a food and a nutritive, cleansing tonic. In the Summer months, small, delicate white flowers cluster and dangle like earrings. Her medicinal seeds can be eaten and pressed for oil, her root harvested in the Fall.

HERBAL & MEDICINAL PROPERTIES

- Nutritive, nourishing herb: full of vitamins, minerals, enzymes.
- Tonic: building new tissue, revitalizing, healing, replenishing
- Beauty herb: building to hair, nails, and skin
- Foundational medicine: where we begin and a safe go-to for all ages after surgery, injury, or illness for healing, replenishing, and nourishing the body
- Digestive system tonic: aids in absorption of nutrients
- Cleansing: supports organs of elimination
- Kidney tonic: diuretic, cleansing to the urinary tract
- Nerve tonic: healing to the adrenals, grounding, calming, energizing.
- Circulatory system tonic: supports the cardiovascular system
- Anti-inflammatory, anti-allergen, strengthening to the immune system
- Antirheumatic, used topically to beat inflamed joints.
- Antiprostatic: used for enlarged prostates
- Menstrual/pregnancy herb: regulating to menses and hormones, building blood, nutritive for pregnancy, postpartum, menopause, lactation

PLANT SPIRIT HEALING

Nettle is a gateway herb for the Green Witch, weaving us back into the fabric of all inside of us and in the Earth that is wild, vital, and free. The first drink of a strong, cold overnight infusion satiates a primordial thirst for deep nourishment that often the cells and soul did not even know they had until then. This grounds the spirit, releasing tension from the physical and emotional body, allowing fear and tightness in the root chakra to dissolve. Thus, we become more grounded, able to bring in nourishment and Earth energy into the body. With daily use, we notice how different we are when we are flooded with nourishment, our basic needs met, our heart open, the taste for wildness and aliveness igniting our spirit, joy and sense of self. The sacral chakra and water element are nourished, the solar plexus, digestive system, and center of courage are awakened, and we begin to exercise better boundaries—finding more clarity and ease in communicating our yes and our no. Nettle is unapologetic, feisty, deeply loving, and wild. It can give us a good talking-to if we are not advocating for ourselves or the Earth, or if we are unbalanced, giving our energy away and becoming depleted. It's a powerful ally for caretakers, healers, mothers, creators, and those who seek to strengthen their communication and mind. Once an ally, nettles becomes foundational, an ally forever.

FAVORITE USES

- Overnight infusion of dried or fresh herb in cold water (drink for a month or more)
- Food medicine: Cook with nettles as with spinach—try nettle quiche, soup, or pesto
- Add leftover nettles from tea to the garden and compost
- Make a second hot infusion with leftover plant material for a hair rinse

OTHER USES

- Fiber for cloth and paper
- Spells of protection
- Natural dye
- Activator for compost, regenerating the Earth; nettle tea for soil

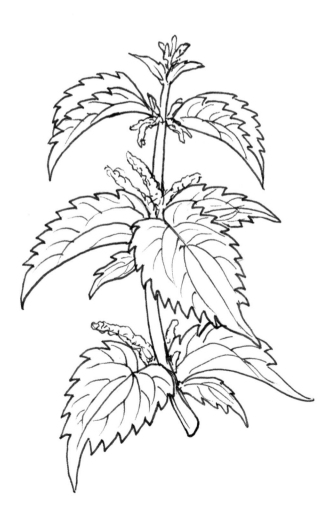

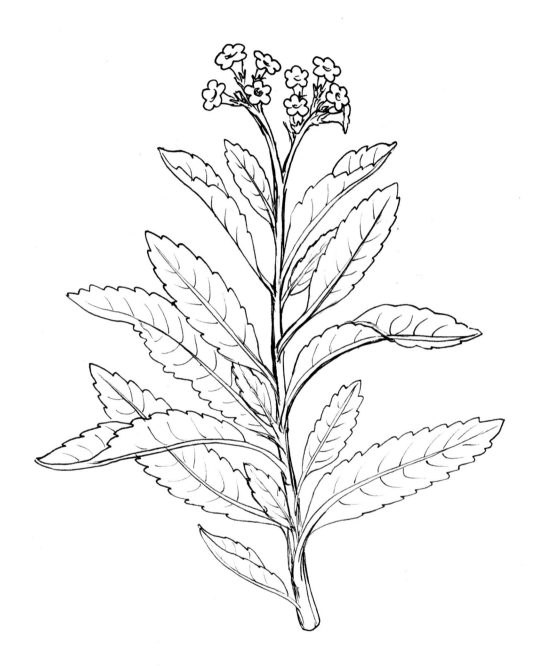

plant profile
Yerba Santa

LATIN NAME *Eriodictyon californicum*

FAMILY Boraginaceae, subfamily Hydrophyllaceae (waterleaf subfamily)

This perennial sticky, shiny, dark-green shrub is native to California, Oregon, and Northern Mexico and lives on dry, sunny mountain slopes. It grows to about the height of a human; its long, serrated, tapered leaves are resinous, leathery, and dark; and it has a surprisingly beautiful panicle of small, purple flowers appearing in late Spring. You can find this ally of the sun and air in wild places where the dust of the desert coats its leaves. After a wildfire went through the land near me, yerba santa was one of the first plants to come back, rejuvenated, rebirthed, bright, vigorous, larger, and healthier then I had ever seen. A couple years later, these patches thrive, renewed.

HERBAL AND MEDICINAL PROPERTIES

- Expectorant: incredible ally for lung and respiratory infections; promotes coughing up of mucous and release of deep, stagnant dark energy

- Bronchodilator and decongestant: opens up breath and air passageways; ally for seasonal allergies and asthma

- Highly aromatic: the bitterness and pungency of yerba santa act as a carminative, helping with digestion

- Antimicrobial: the essential oils kill microbes and have a cleansing and purifying effect on the mucous membranes and body

- Used for thousands of years by the Native people of its lands; the name yerba santa means "holy herb" and suggests it was used for a variety of ailments.

- I enjoy mixing this herb with my smoke blends, feeling how it opens up my breath and lungs with its lovely aroma.

- The plant speaks to me in meditations about using her for oral health; I often find myself rubbing her leaves along my gums when I am hiking, and I can feel how this increases circulation around my teeth and is cleansing

PLANT SPIRIT HEALING

Yerba santa grounds the spirit, calming the nervous system, quieting the mind, and opening the breath. This quality makes the plant spirit a wonderful ally for meditation and shamanic journeying. It also goes deep into dark places, illuminating shadows while holding the nervous system in peace and loving support. Darkness dissolves, and I am often shown what is being healed or how to remedy a situation. The resinous, purifying oils coat my throat and insides as I drink him in, opening my breath, lungs, and heart. This plant spirit brings the gift of purification, peace, and quiet while shifting consciousness, helping us access deeper states of consciousness and meditation and opening the third eye and crown chakra from a grounded, still, rooted place.

FAVORITE USES

- Hot tea for colds, lung infections, and meditation

- With mullein in an herbal smoke blend

- As a honey or alcohol/honey elixir

- As an ingredient in cough syrup

- To rub on the teeth and gums for oral hygiene in the wilderness

- To sit with in the wild, appreciating its grounding, calming, and beautiful presence

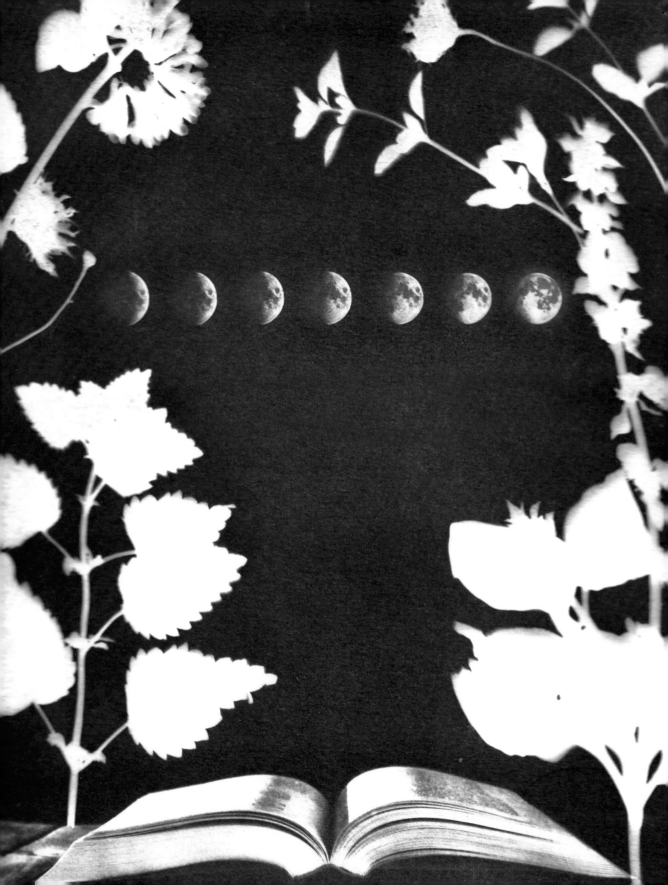

EAST PORTAL JOURNAL PROMPTS

Reflect on the element of air in you.

Air element in balance

- Great imagination, visioning, and intelligence balanced with the grounded ability to bring dreams into manifested form (balanced with earth)

- Open-mind balanced with knowing yourself and good boundaries (balanced with fire)

- Ability to think and feel in a balanced way (balanced with water)

Air element out of balance

- Being scattered, flighty, inconsistent, uncommitted, or forgetful (needs more earth)

- Anxiety, nervousness, or paranoia (needs more earth and balanced fire)

- Excessive multitasking, being involved in too many projects, inability to focus on one thing (needs more earth)

- Unable to feel emotions and be with the feelings in the body, wanting to explain things away (needs more water)

Close your eyes and call in your inner child or Maiden archetype.

Reflect on how you can nourish your inner Maiden archetype in your journal:

- How can you cultivate more spontaneous play? Make a list of play dates you want to have with yourself or others. Put them in your calendar. Make them happen!

- How can you put yourself in the right time and place for an adventure?

- What would be fun?

- What does your inner child love?

- Create a vision board for your year, your dream career, home, life, or the like. What other playful, creative, or practical ways can you vision, dream into, and plan for your future?

- What are some new habits you would like to incorporate into your way of moving through the world? How can you start with baby steps and grow into that full expression?

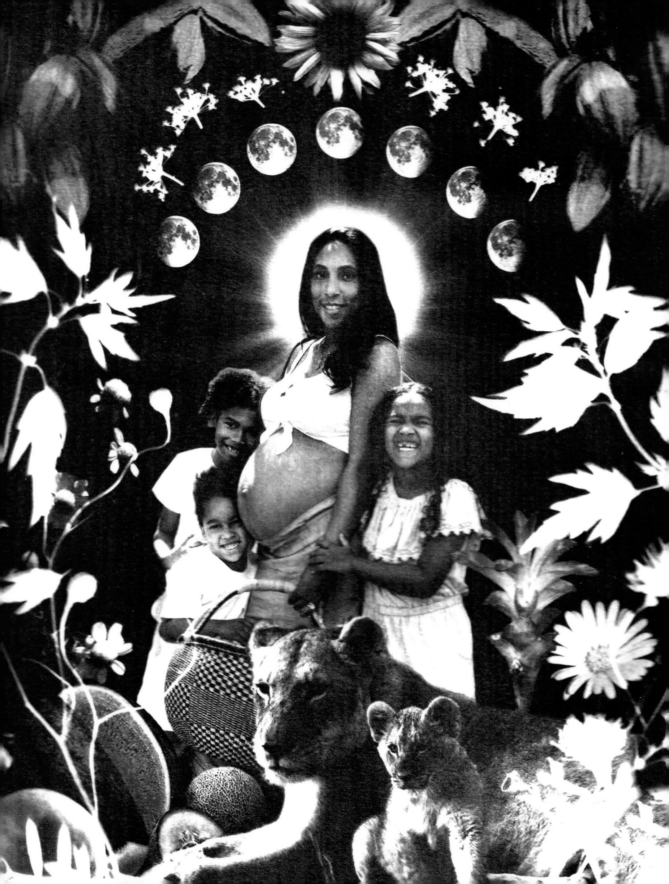

Chapter 5

Earth Magick and Medicine of Summer

Ripen & Thrive: Action & Transformation | South · Fire · The Mother

The Portal of the South at a Glance

ELEMENT Fire

TIME OF DAY Midday | 10:00 a.m.–4:00 p.m.

MOON PHASE Full

SEASON OF SOLAR YEAR Summer | June, July, August

EARTH HOLY DAYS Litha (Summer Solstice/ Midsummer) | June 19–23

WHEEL OF LIFE ARCHETYPE Mother | Age 21–41

ENERGIES Growing, expanding, nurturing, doing, transforming, creating, taking care of others, responsibility, accountability, mothering, networking, moving energy, alchemy, being out in the public, planning for an abundant future, working hard, becoming more resilient, taking risks, practicing courage

HEALING HERBS

Circulatory tonics Hawthorn berry, rosemary, lemon balm, cacao, cinnamon

Strengthening/uplifting/antidepressant herbs Rhodiola, schisandra, Saint John's wort, lemon balm

Demulcent herbs Calendula, marshmallow, comfrey, slippery elm

Digestive tonics Nourishing herbs, adaptogens, bitters, carminatives, spices

Nourishing herbs and adaptogens Nettles, chickweed, burdock, schisandra, eleuthero

TENDING THE GARDEN Greatest amount of work required in the garden: consistent harvesting, weeding, trimming, composting, mulching, watering, tending; abundance of medicine to harvest, tincture, dry, preserve; the more we work in the garden in the summer, the more food and medicine is generated

APOTHECARY Harvesting and making medicine, making tinctures from fresh plants and dry herbs, infusing honeys

RITUALS Rituals of celebration, community, abundance, generosity, harvest, transformation, fire, empowerment, and rites of passage

Gaia speaks

Full are my baskets,
ripe are my fruits,
hot is the sweltering sun on my skin.

Drip goes my sweat.
Love from my heart
nourishes creations, land, and kin.

I give and I take,
circulate energy and grow
power within,
above, and below.

The cauldron of iron,
round like the full moon,
the fire inside
fuels courage and truth

In power I rise,
transforming all in my sight,
make medicine from poison,
receiving the nourishment from life.

I expand and I do,
responsible and true.
Empowered I act,
my being a gift, dripping juice like ripe fruit.

Now is my time.
Eat me and I'll eat you.
I birth, work, transform.
From seed I grow food.

There's a revolution in me
fueled by passion and clarity.
Though I'm woven in responsibility,
I bend the laws of time and space
and thus beyond what you see
I know I am truly free.

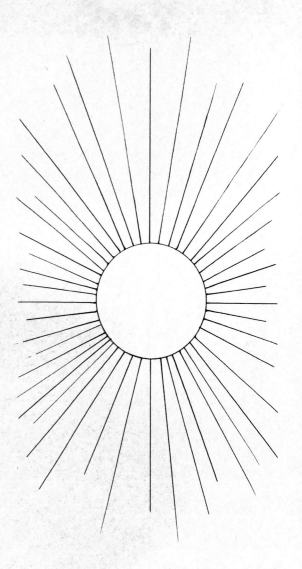

Ripen to Regenerate Yourself, Life-Giving Mother

Summer! The peak of solar expression, the longest days of the year, the time when sweat drips down our brow, our hearts beat hot, and we cool ourselves with hydrating gifts from our abundant gardens, including raw salads, cucumbers, and fruit. On these long days, it is hard to remember when the full sun was just being born on the other side of the wheel at the Winter Solstice. He was just a babe then, so meek, so in need of encouragement. He grew through the Spring of our youth, and even those days feel far away when we find ourselves melting in the strength and light of the solar rays. Now we seek shade, moments of rest, and tall glasses of cold drinks. And yet, our enthusiasm is ripe, there is much to be done in the garden, our lives feel full, and projects are riding the currents of their own momentum.

Now is the time of the Mother archetype: she who feeds all the children, multitasks, and moves miraculous amounts of energy. Those of us who are mothers know how motherhood stretches us beyond what we thought we were capable of. There is not enough time in the day, and yet the archetypal Mother tends to her children, creates life, mothers, encourages, feeds, and supports. Even if we don't have human children, we can relate to this archetype if we have birthed a business or project. In the Spring of birthing a new creation into being, we never expect the amount of work, effort, and labor we must pour forth when the energy climaxes in its portal of Summer. Somehow, through the expansive energy we circulate, through the transformative fire element of the portal of South, we ourselves are re-created. We often surpass our own expectations as we ride a regenerative current in peak expression. Sometimes we feel we are just along for the ride, working hard to keep up. Riding these high currents, we often stumble, fall, and have to pick ourselves up again. When we do, we become more resilient and wise—we grow up. Our efforts at this time must be to ride these powerful waves without burning out, midwifing our own deaths, rebirths, and transformations, and mothering the Mother (ourselves).

In the garden, the seeds that incubated in the darkness of Winter womb and that we tenderly planted with prayers in the Spring are now unrecognizable. They are in full bounty, glory, and wild abundance. The food garden is exploding with tomatoes, squash, herbs, and flowers. When I lived in Vermont, we laughed in awe at the ridiculous abundance a few seeds created, and we secretly left the never-ending surplus of squash at one another's doorsteps or at the side of the road with a "free" sign. In the heat of the Summer months, Gaia gifts us with an abundance of hydrating and cooling food and herbs to help us balance the yang energies of the summer with yin produce such as cucumbers, watermelon, mint, salads, and other fruits and veggies.

The seasons of Spring and Summer are Earth's exhale. The expansive energy of this portal has the plants growing out toward the sun and moving their life force into flower, fruit, and seed production. In biodynamic gardening, we tend to these places where the plants meet the air and sun with practices such as foliar and atmospheric sprays or plant teas.

Our medicinal garden, too, is at its peak of production, pollination, and expression. Like the Mother archetype, the garden's Earth body is deeply interwoven in a humming, ever transforming ecosystem in peak alchemy. Bees, butterflies, insects, and birds are all riding the expansive energies of our perennial plants. The long days of Summer make it an ideal time to garden. Nature encourages us to spend hours outside each day, harvesting flowers to dry or make

into medicine, cutting back herbs, composting, and weeding where necessary. The more we touch the herbs, take from and give to them, the more abundance is generated in the garden. Like all beings in reciprocal relationships, plants being cultivated produce more food, are healthier, and thrive better than those left on their own. And so, our medicine gardens teach us about the alchemy of moving great transformative energy through our bodies and the land we love, where we reap the medicine and magick of reciprocity and relationship.

The energy we move and the work we do now in ourselves, our communities, and the lands we tend will lead to a rich harvest, a magickal apothecary, and much to be grateful for in the Fall. Herbal raw juices, demulcent teas, cold nourishing herb infusions, and iced teas of hibiscus and schisandra, rich in vitamin C, keep us energized, cool, hydrated, and balanced. Otherwise, the high solar energy can lead to burnout if we ride them to an extreme.

The South's portals of thriving open to you at the climax of each energy cycle in nature. We are supported in moving the greatest amount of energy each day at noon, each full moon, each Summer season, and in the peak years of your career and life. Draw from the deep roots you sent into the regenerative darkness of the Earth's soil in seasons past. Fill yourself from the source of all life force energy—from the depths of the Earth, from your roots, pulling Earth energy into your replenished adrenals, nourished nervous system, and renewed immune system. Expand with the exhalation of the Earth, reaching out like the plants, growing toward the radiant sun. Be bold; shine bright; play, work, generate in the ripe fullness of an unapologetic you. Now is the time! Don't hesitate—shine!

Ripen to regenerate yourself, life-giving Mother.

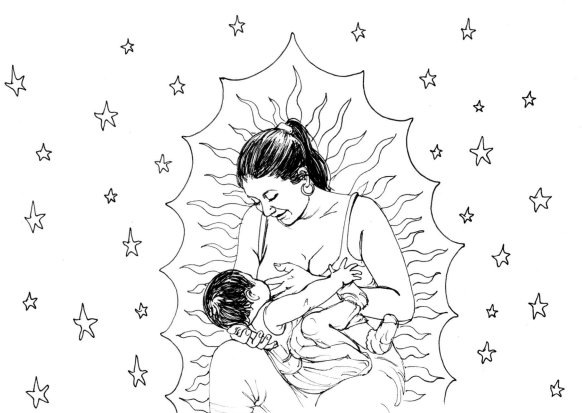

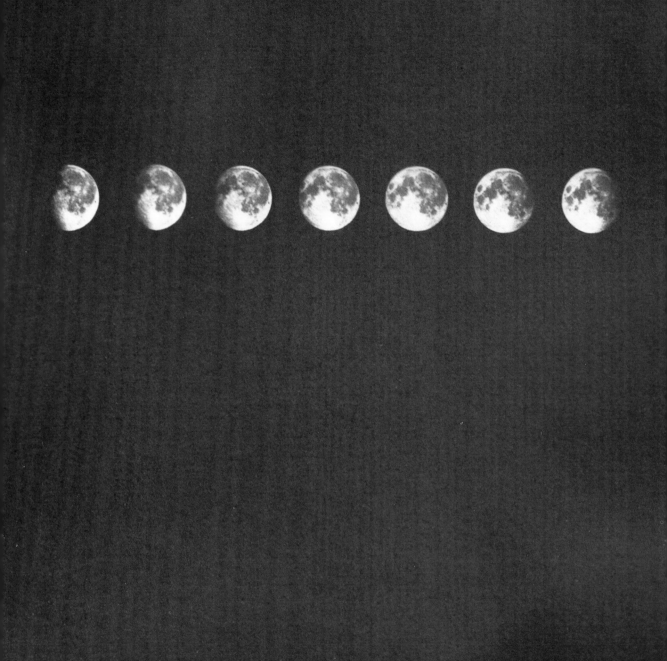

Entering the Portals of the South

The portal of the South is a current of climactic energy that we ride in the middle part of the day, at the full moon, in the summertime, and in the prime of our lives.

In the night sky, the full moon is the peak of the lunar cycle in full expression. We celebrate under the light of the moon, giving gratitude for the prayers we cast with the new moon. We acknowledge what we have received and what has come to fruition with grateful hearts. The full moon is an ideal time for gatherings, prayer circles, rituals, moon bathing, meditation, manifesting, and relaxing in awe and wonder. At times, the energy of the full moon is ecstatic—perfect for being naked outside in the moonlight, for spells, lovemaking, and riding waves of wildness. Other times, the full moon can make us feel like "lunatics"—and then balancing the energy with yin practices that belong to the portal of the dark moon help us harmonize and stay centered. On those occasions, solitude, reflection, journaling, ritual baths, meditation, sound baths (see page 204), rest, intuitive art making, and being more still outside can be very healing.

In the menstrual cycle, ovulation corresponds with the full moon. Herbs, foods, and practices that encourage circulation in the womb help us have a healthy cycle. It is a wonderful time to practice vaginal steaming, as it encourages circulation and movement of chi in the womb—unless you wish to conceive or already have, in which case vaginal steaming is not advisable.

On our Wheel of the Year, the season of Summer spans the months of June, July, and August in the Northern Hemisphere, with the Summer Solstice (June 19–23) marking the official start of Summer, the longest day of the year, the peak of solar expression. After this, the energy of the year will slowly wane, the heat continuing but the nights growing in length. Midway between the Summer Solstice and the Fall Equinox, we celebrate the cross-quarter holiday of Lughnasadh, or Lammas, on August 1. It is the first harvest festival, honoring the mature aspect of the Sun God. It is the time when the grains are harvested. By celebrating each of the three harvest festivals, humans weave their gratitude and strengthen the life-force energy that continues to feed and bring abundance.

In the wheel of our lives, Summer corresponds to the archetype of the Mother and our "adulthood," roughly ages twenty-one to forty-two. This transformative time is when we truly grow up—becoming wiser and more resilient through the trials of life. We become more expansive and capable, stretching ourselves, throwing ourselves passionately into projects, creations, community, or family. Many times, we burn out and thus learn how to mother ourselves and sustain our energy. We often refine our purpose, deepen our relationships with community, create a career, and perhaps start a family. The expansiveness, curiosity, exploration, and experiments of our youth—the time of the Maiden archetype—may now be channeled in productive ways, though part of running such high-fire energy is learning to get burned along the way, to heal, recover, transform and begin anew. We are often pushed beyond what we thought we were capable of. In this portal, we often learn to heal heartbreak, sit with pain, be unafraid of suffering, and face challenges with courage, knowing they will transform us and we will grow. This is our time to be bold, take risks, and grow in strength and power. This portal ends at age forty-two, a time that tends to be accompanied by a "midlife crisis," with regrets and doubts about having lived life fully or succeeded in certain areas. Perhaps throwing ourselves courageously into the transformative fires of the South helps us arrive in completion and readiness for the waning of the West.

RIDING THE CURRENTS OF THE SOUTH DURING THE DAY

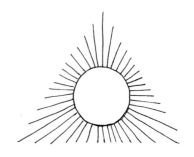

In the twenty-four-hour wheel of the day, South corresponds to middle of the day, roughly from 10:00 a.m. to 4:00 p.m. This is the most "yang" time of the day, warmest and brightest, with the strongest energy. Our bodies, interwoven into the fabric of all of nature, mirror this. Thus, many cultures traditionally eat the largest meal at noon—the time when our digestive fire is also strongest.

Because the solar energy within and around us is at its peak, this is the most suitable time of the day to be productive, to move the greatest transformative energy while staying in balance. We can crescendo our energy at 10:00 and enter a highly productive flow, take a lunch break, pause and digest, and go back into an afternoon flow that begins to wane at 4:00. However, if we need to work a more traditional work schedule that extends on either side, it is especially beneficial to take breaks during our day. In many Latin cultures, the hottest part of the workday, after lunch, is reserved for a siesta—a nap. Thus, in the middle of the most solar time of the day, the energies are brought into balance by calling upon the tools of the North and rest. In northern climates, where the days are not as long or hot during most of the year, this is not the custom.

In the Summer portal, we learn how to modulate our nervous system so we do not burn out. In the course of the day this means focusing on one thing at a time, taking breaks, moving the body and stretching, staying hydrated, and getting some fresh air. If we try to push our minds, bodies, and creativity into a linear pattern or push productivity with coffee, sugar, or other stimulants, we eventually get off the regenerative tracks, deplete our system, and burn out. Ride the energies of this portal following smaller spiral flows of energy,

renewing yourself many times in the larger arc of creative output. Taking two minutes to close your eyes and breathe in between tasks, or to sit on the Earth outside for ten minutes, increases your productivity and regenerates your mind and energy.

The portal of the South connects us to the fire in our belly, our digestive system and our solar plexus. Physically, this is an opportunity to notice if your fire is low, in which case you may feel sluggish, depressed, lethargic, unmotivated, or sad. You may have slow digestion, get bloating from eating, or feel tired. If you have excess fire, you may have a high metabolism and difficulty absorbing nutrients from your food. You may experience blood-sugar drops, "hanger" (anger or moodiness caused by hunger), anxiety, scattered thoughts, and ungroundedness. If your fire is in balance, you have a steady, warm, and joyful disposition and a positive outlook. You feel motivated, engaged, enthusiastic, passionate, and optimistic. You can enjoy a meal without anxiety and enjoy a pause without rushing yourself or feeling chaotic. This state of harmony is what allows us to thrive and what Nature shows us leads to longevity. Notice how you can support your fire to experience balance each day.

Daily Practices to Balance Your Fire Element

If your fire element is low, activate it with any of these practices:

- Movement, including yoga, cardio, or boxing

- Five to ten minutes of sun salutations to move energy

- Inversion—standing on your head, hanging upside down, getting blood into your brain, and moving your lymph

- Warming elixirs and herbs that increase circulation, such as ginger, rosemary, cacao, turmeric, thyme, schisandra berry, or hawthorn

- Warm foods like blended soups and bone broth, which are easy to digest—avoid cold and damp "yin" foods and drinks, such as raw foods, salads, or ice water

- Taking an herbal bitter twenty minutes before a meal to assist with digestion

- Drinking ginger, peppermint, or another digestive tea after a meal

- Drinking espresso or green tea, or eating cacao, especially if blood pressure is low and if your constitution agrees with it, in moderation

- Taking a walk outside

- Avoiding snacking too much between meals—allow each meal to fully digest so you do not dampen your digestive fire

- Practicing the Breath of Fire yoga technique

If your fire element is overcharged, bring balance with yin practices such as:

- Staying hydrated

- Drinking cool, moist herbs, such as marshmallow, jasmine, white peony root, linden, chickweed, motherwort, or dandelion leaf

- Eating raw veggies and fruit

- Eating grounding snacks with healthy fats

- Using rose spray or another mist made with water and cooling essential oils, such as peppermint

- Breathing, meditating, and calming the nervous system

- Creating a relaxing environment

- Listening to meditative and calming music

- Taking baths, doing self-massage, or oiling the skin

- Practicing yoga, swimming, or tai chi, choosing movement that is centering and grounding to the spirit

What Is True Power?

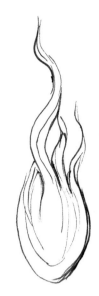

Power can be a trigger word for the modern empath because to our current culture, it means having power over *someone else, something, or some place. This is not true power but domination, control, oppression, entanglement, and sickness.*

True power is the ability to transform anything.

It is something we cultivate in the soul, in the flame of the solar plexus. We do this through right action, courage, unapologetically loving ourselves, and walking in devotion and right relationship as we are guided by the mysterious whispers of the Great Mystery and the stirrings in our hearts and souls.

The ability to transform comes from stretching ourselves, taking risks, being brave, confronting injustice, facing truth, and diving into the fire of transformation. With true power, we are not afraid of life. We do not turn away from all the flavors that are inevitably part of being human. We rejoice in sweetness but also accept, receive, and learn to digest the pain, the bitter flavors, the challenges, and the traumas.

The digestive system is a perfect metaphor for the role of the fire element that resides in the corresponding solar plexus chakra. A healthy digestive system allows us to eat all sorts of foods and turn matter into energy to grow and regenerate. Once we have taken from our food what we can use, the rest is meant to be released through our bowels—out of our bodies for good! If we do not release it, it gets reabsorbed by the membranes of the colon back into our blood, causing toxicity and illness.

This is exactly what happens when we do not fully process the challenges and traumas of life. We must radically face the truth of what life has served us, and we must be bold and courageous, having faith in our fire—in our ability to transform the experiences of life into fuel or waste to be released. We digest them, transforming them into medicine we can absorb for our growth and evolution. We ask ourselves, "What is the medicine in this situation, illness, or relationship?" We find the gift, the nourishment in all that greets us, receiving it, allowing it to change us and help us grow. And the rest? We release it from our energetic and physical bodies, cleansing our hearts, returning it to the Earth Mother to be transformed into compost.

Everything contains some food for growth and evolution. Life is here to change us. Don't hide from transformation; it is inevitable, and your courage will help your power grow. As your power grows, your confidence increases, and you will realize that you truly can transform anything and everything. That includes yourself, over and over, again and again.

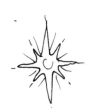

CELEBRATING WITH THE FULL MOON

One day a month, the moon swells in her luminous fullness in the dark night sky. Celebrate this night as holy. Create pause to spend time with her, drink her in. Moon bathing is the practice of receiving her light into your body—much like suntanning. You can expose your genitals to the moonlight and feel the moonlight entering your sacred womb or sacral charka, your fertile void, your yin spaces. Cleanse your crystals and charge them in the moonlight (see page 62).

The full moon is a time when Witches gather for rituals, celebrations, and spell casting. Some full moons have a social energy and are a wonderful time to connect with your sacred friends, share a meal, and go for a walk in the moonlight. You can cast a circle together under the light and say some prayers. The simple practice of gathering with dear friends each full moon and new moon has a powerful effect in aligning your body to the rhythms of nature. It's also an organic way of creating a coven of sorts—a sacred container for prayer, ritual, and sharing from the heart.

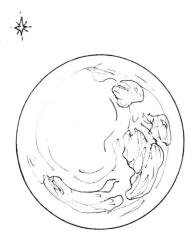

Some full moons have a "lunatic" or chaotic energy. In those cases, you can draw on the practices of the dark moon—solitude, meditation, ritual baths, and alone time in nature—to balance the energies if they are feeling too expansive, or if you are feeling uncentered.

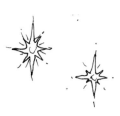

THE MOTHER ARCHETYPE

The healthy mother is herself mothered. The thriving mother is interwoven in a village or a community of reciprocal support. At this time in our lives, we move so much energy, creating and giving of ourselves, that we may become depleted if we are isolated or alone. We simply cannot access the immensity of energy available in the Great Web when we are not interconnected in a web of support. No wonder so many mothers have postpartum depression, overwhelmed by the challenges, changes, responsibilities, demands, and lack of experience of becoming a new mother. No wonder so many new business owners burn out, feeling isolated and alone or as part of a competitive culture instead of a collaborative culture.

In the abundant Summer garden, the bees, flowers, soil, worms, birds, thunderclouds, rains, sunflowers, gardeners, children playing, and cats napping are one organism, thriving and living in giving and receiving. May we learn from the thriving garden and create thriving communities of mutual support and collaboration where each individual's success is seen as a benefit to all.

In the Summer, we celebrate Independence Day in the United States. Let us start celebrating our interdependence instead. Let us acknowledge all who participated in our growth and expansion, knowing we never accomplish anything on our own. Let us share in the wealth of this energy, understanding the laws of alchemy and magick, in which the whole is greater than the sum of its parts. Let us throw the old cultures of competing, individuation, superstardom, domination, and hierarchy into the cauldrons of transformation. Let us gather in circle under the full moon's light as equals, as one. Let us thrive.

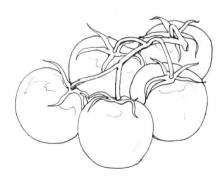

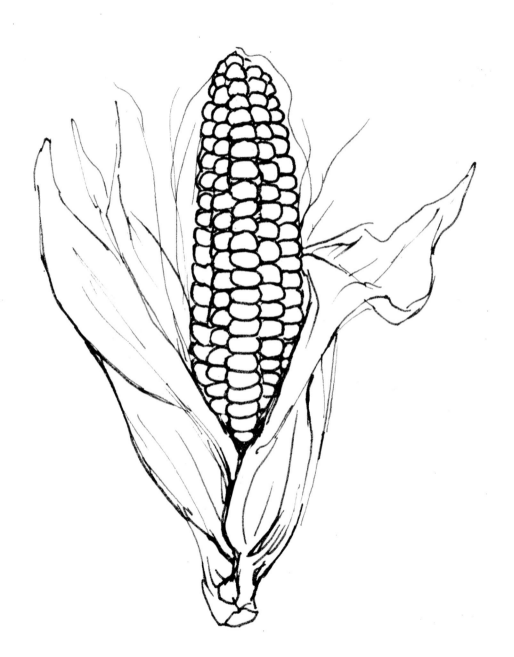

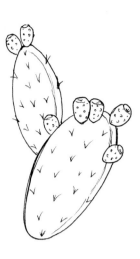

EARTH MEDICINE OF THE SOUTH: ACTIVATION AND HYDRATION

The fire element is the quickest to change, and it can be volatile. It is the element Witches work with to create the greatest transformation in the shortest amount of time. All elements hold the power of change, but fire can quickly transform great matter into nothing but ash.

For this reason, when working with the fire element in the portal of the South, we work with plants and practices that help us stay in balance. Balance is an active state; just like healing is a lifelong journey of unending growth and transformation, balance is not an end goal or a destination we reach. When we see someone walking a tightrope, we notice that balance requires constant awareness, presence, and attention. A breeze nudges us from one side, and we respond right away to stay in balance.

The medicinal plants that support us in the South portal embody the diverse aspects of the fire element. Some, such as ginger or cayenne, awaken our fire and can make us burn quick and hot. Others, such as lemon balm or calendula, soothe the fire element in us while supporting the light of our inner flame. Demulcent herbs, such as marshmallow, slippery elm, and licorice root, can cool, heal, and repair tissue that has been burned; they are anti-inflammatory, calming excess heat in the body.

In the portal of the South, we work to support the movement of our energy and blood with circulatory-system tonics such as hawthorn berry, ginger, turmeric, rosemary, mint, cacao, and culinary herbs. We

strengthen our sense of power and joy with adaptogens and antidepressant herbs such as rhodiola, schisandra, Saint John's wort, and lemon balm. We support our ability to transform food with digestive system tonics made from nourishing herbs (see pages 54 to 55) and herbal bitters (see pages 80 to 81). We raise our energy with adaptogens and stimulants such as cacao, mate, tea, schisandra, and rhodiola. We cool our bodies with herbs that lower our temperature and remove heat, including dandelion leaves, herbs in the mint family, and linden leaf and flower. We stay nourished and grounded with nourishing herbs, which restore our adrenals and replenish the systems that are working hard. We calm our spirit with spiritually centering herbs such as tulsi, reishi, and motherwort, which bring the wisdom and inner silence associated with the dark-moon North portal. They can be balancing when the fires of the South portal begin to feel overwhelming or chaotic.

We can support the activation, balancing, and hydration with food medicine as well.

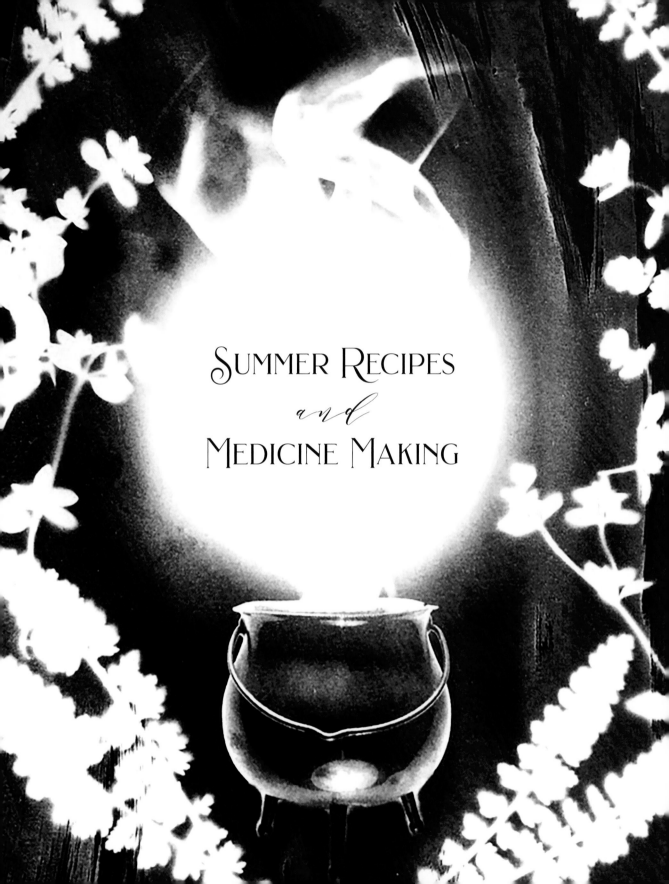

SUMMER RECIPES

and

MEDICINE MAKING

The overnight nourishing herb infusions described in the Spring portal (see page 55) are a staple to our tradition of herbal healing year around. Continuing to work with your daily wild-weed ally will keep you grounded and nourished with replenished adrenals during the busy Summer months. And while the Wise Woman tradition tends to favor overnight infusions as the primary method of intaking herbs, Summer is a great time to expand our apothecary and medicine-making methods. Following are some other methods herbalists use to extract plant medicine.

Tinctures

What's the difference between a tea, an infusion, and a tincture? A tea is created by steeping any plant in hot water for about twenty minutes. An infusion is steeped for a minimum of four hours. The longer time extracts a greater amount of minerals, vitamins, and other alkaloids. Drinking infusions helps us develop a deeper sensitivity to the plant we are working with. It is easy to self-dose as you drink sip by sip, noticing how much of an herb you need that day. Infusions are also nourishing and easy to assimilate into the body. Taking an herbal capsule, on the other hand, is a commitment to a set dose, even though plants have different effects on different people. A tincture is an alcohol extraction of an herb. It is concentrated, strong medicine, diluted in water for consuming.

For some purposes, tinctures are preferable. First, it takes a lot of plant material to make an infusion. The same amount tinctured in alcohol makes enough medicine to last many moons for many more people. When working with medicine that uses ingredients less abundant than wild weeds, this factor of sustainability is reason enough. Second, alcohol extractions make stronger medicine, which is sometimes better for acute conditions. Third, adding two to three drops of tincture to a few ounces of water is simple, easy to remember, and great for people on the go or traveling. I always travel with a 1-ounce (30 ml) tincture of an antimicrobial herb, such as white sage, usnea, or yerba santa—it can easily kick bacteria I may be exposed to on my travels before they take hold. Finally, tinctures capture a moment in time of a plant's expression and your connection. If you have a relationship with a particular herb or place, create ceremony in harvesting, perhaps doing it on a holy Earth day. All of that is woven into the medicine you make. When you can take that medicine, you reexperience the magick of that never-to-be-repeated moment in time. For instance, I have a tincture of Saint John's wort that I made in ecstatic ceremony on the Summer Solstice in a field in Poland with the moon in Leo. Each drop of that potion is a full body *yes* of solar magick!

Fresh Leaf Tincture

In the summer, many medicinal herbs used for their aerial parts (often the leaf and flower) are at their peak of vitality and ready to be harvested. The folk method of making herbal tinctures is quite simple and foolproof.

Yield: varies

> Herb to harvest*
> 80- to 100-proof organic vodka, brandy, mezcal, or other alcohol of your choice (to be shelf stable, menstruum must be at least 25 percent alcohol, or 50 proof)

1. Create sacred space.

2. Harvest the herb with intention, using the sacred harvesting method (see pages 34 to 35).

3. Loosely chop the plant material and fill any size jar about 90 percent full without stuffing it or making it too compact.

4. Pour your menstruum over the herbs.

5. Ensure the plant material is fully submerged; if not, push it down with a utensil. Cover the jar.

6. Label your medicine. Keep it away from direct sunlight, and shake it every once in a while.

7. Strain and bottle after two months or more.

*If you are using dried plant material, you will use one-third the amount as fresh—so your jar will be about one-third full instead of 90 percent full before you add your menstruum.

Herb-Infused Honey

Herb-infused honeys are pure bliss—medicine of delight! The honey gently extracts the medicinal properties of the herbs and is particularly wonderful for aromatic herbs, such as sage, tulsi, or lemon balm, or for flowers. A sage honey is wonderful to have in your apothecary for cold Winter months, when a spoon of it in hot water will make an instant fresh antibacterial tea and will bring you into the delight of the summer months while helping you fight flu symptoms. You can also cook and bake with your herbal honeys, spread them on toast, eat them by the spoonful, add them to elixirs . . . you get the idea.

Yield: varies

> Herb to harvest*
> Raw honey

1. Create sacred space.

2. Harvest the herb with intention, using the sacred harvesting method (see pages 34 to 35).

3. Loosely chop the plant material and fill a jar of any size about 90 percent full without stuffing it or making it too compact.

4. Pour the honey over the herbs. Use a chopstick or spoon to get bubbles out.

5. Label your medicine. Keep it away from direct sunlight, and shake it every once in a while.

6. Strain and bottle after two months or more.

*If you are using dried plant material, you will use one-third the amount as fresh—so your jar will be about one-third full instead of 90 percent full before you add your honey.

Peace and Bliss Tincture

This is my lovely formula for easing stress and anxiety and to bring the mind, nervous system, and air element into balance. The milky oats holy basil and skullcap are restorative to the nervous system and adrenals, and the blend is aromatic, opening the breath and heart, calming the belly, and centering the mind.

Yield: varies

> 1 part holy basil
> 1 part oat straw or milky oat tops
> 1 part skullcap
> Organic vodka

1. If using dried herbs, fill a jar of any size one-third with equal amounts of each one. If using fresh herbs, blend in the vodka after making sure your fresh herbs fill your container.

2. Bottle, let the mixture sit for at least two months, shaking periodically, and strain.

3. Add 1 teaspoon (5 ml) to ¼ cup (60 ml) of water and drink two or three times a day, or when feeling stressed.

Love Potion

This love potion draws on the heat of passion, the plants of the tropics, and the prayers in your heart! Take each ingredient and pray into it, calling forth the spirit of the plant and the qualities you ask it to bring to your medicine.

Yield: varies

> ½ jar's worth fresh passion-vine leaves, vine, and perhaps a flower for sensuality, flow, creativity, and self-love
> 1 fresh rose for the highest vibration of unconditional love and grace
> 1 stick cinnamon for passion and spicy sweetness—sparks that fly!
> 1 thumb-size piece fresh ginger for heat and moving sacral waters
> ¼ jar dried damiana herb for a relaxed, warm, fluid flow
> 1 handful dried hawthorn berries for a courageous, strong, loving heart
> Generous amount raw honey for the bees, alchemists, pollinators, and lovers
> Splash of Flora Sagrada Rose hydrosol— sacred Bulgarian roses for ancient, timeless love
> 1 stick of vanilla for sweet, safe pleasure
> Rum or another alcohol of your choice, such as tequila or brandy

1. Combine all the plant ingredients in a glass jar of any size with a lid and top it off with the alcohol.

2. Shake with prayers and spells. Seal with the lid, label, and allow it to sit for at least two months, shaking periodically.

3. Strain and add to hot cocoa, elixirs, teas, raw chocolate, or Lovers' Licking Chocolate (see page 126).

Fresh Herbal Juices

We learned the "herstory" behind fresh herbal juices (see Raw Herbal Juices, page 81) and some great spring juice recipes. Following are my favorite herbal juices for the summer months, keeping us hydrated and cool.

Nerve-Repair Mint, Comfrey, and Saint John's Juice

This is one of my all-time favorite fresh juices. It is delicious, refreshing, and hydrating. Everyone loves it! The predominant flavor of fresh mint makes it a desirable form of nutritive replenishment on a hot summer day. The other medicinal herbs, comfrey and Saint John's wort, are incredible allies for supporting cellular, tissue, and nerve regeneration in the body.

Be aware that not all herbalists agree about using comfrey internally—some insist it is unsafe, and many herbalists get into heated debates on the topic. Other herbalists drink comfrey on a regular basis and question the methods of researching the toxicity of some alkaloids in the plant. I adore comfrey and find it to be one of my most beloved allies and healers, though I do not consume or recommend consuming it daily for an extended period of time, such as a few months. However, in my many years of working with comfrey, I have seen it to heal so deeply and profoundly. (For more about comfrey, including several precautions, see pages 210 to 211.)

I shared this recipe with my dear friend Linda, who made this fresh juice five out of seven days a week for a few weeks and experienced a healing of old nerve tissue around her knee from an accident that had taken place six years prior. This is a deeply healing, regenerative juice.

Yield: 1 serving

> 2 handfuls fresh mint leaves
> 1 small fresh comfrey leaf
> 1 handful fresh Saint John's wort leaves

1. Add ingredients to a blender full of spring water.

2. Blend, strain, and serve over ice.

3. Bottle and store in the fridge.

Watermelon-Mint Juice

In the summer, the garden gifts us hydrating fruits and vegetables, which are full of minerals, vitamins, and antioxidants that keep us nourished, cool, and energized. Watermelons are about 90 percent water, and they are a good source of vitamins as well as potassium, copper, and antioxidants. Blended with fresh peppermint and ice, this juice is refreshing, sweet, delicious, awakening, uplifting, and energizing.

Yield: 1 serving

> 4 cups (600 g) fresh watermelon
> 1 cup (96 g) fresh peppermint
> 1 cup (140 g) ice cubes

1. Cut watermelon into cubes, removing rind and seeds.

2. Blend all ingredients and enjoy!

Cooling Iced Teas

Schisandra Infusion

This simple schisandra infusion is the embodied energy of thriving in the full expression, enthusiasm, and expansion of the summer portal. Schisandra is an energizing, stimulating adaptogen, detoxifying to the body, focusing to the mind, and uplifting and empowering to the spirit. Read more about schisandra on pages 136 to 137 and enjoy drinking her to connect to the motivated, creative energy available in the Summer portal.

Yield: 1 quart (946 ml)

> 1 tablespoon (25 g) dried whole schisandra berry (not powder)

1. Infuse the berries in 1 quart (946 ml) of hot water for an hour or more, preferably overnight.

2. As you drink the infusion, feel free to chew and eat the hydrated berries to receive all of her medicinal properties. Enjoy throughout the day to stay energized. A great ally to work with daily for a month to enjoy the maximum benefits of detoxification and activation.

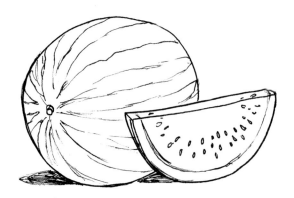

Schisandra-Hibiscus Spritzer

Both schisandra and hibiscus are high in vitamin C, tonify the reproductive system, and hold the essence of thriving sensuality and bright energy. This infusion has a delicious lemony flavor and beautiful fuchsia color. Mixed with carbonated water and an optional sweetener, this effervescent pink drink is uplifting, beautifying, and fun for parties. You can also spike it with a nice vodka for a fabulous cocktail.

Yield: varies

> 1 tablespoon (25 g) dried whole schisandra
>   berry
> 2 tablespoons (3.5 g) dried hibiscus flower
> Sweetener of choice (optional)
> Vodka (optional)

1. Allow the herbs to infuse in 1 quart (946 ml) of hot water for an hour or more.

2. Dilute halfway with sparkling water. May be sweetened or spiked with vodka. Serve over ice. Both the hibiscus flowers and the schizandra berries are edible, so no need to strain.

Goddess Beauty Infusion

This tea is incredibly beautiful—a clear fuschia color. It is also incredibly beautifying, rich in antioxidants, minerals, vitamins, and nutrients. Made of two of my favorite exalted Goddess herbs, butterfly blue pea and schisandra, this blend came through in meditation, where it was revealed that both plants are allies for manifestation, empowered creativity, sensuality, and embodied feminine power together balanced in their yin and yang aspects. Drink daily for a couple of weeks for greatest benefits and results.

Yield: 1 quart (946 ml)

> 1 tablespoon (7 g) dried butterfly blue pea
>   flower
> 1 tablespoon (25 g) whole schisandra berry

1. Steep together in 1 quart (946 ml) of hot water for an hour or longer to make a deeply medicinal, adaptogenic and magickal infusion.

2. Serve over ice during the summer or dilute, to taste.

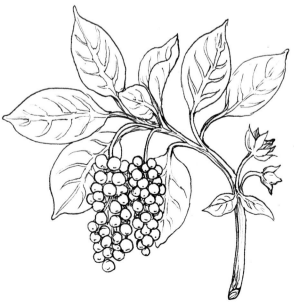

Coffee and Chocolate Creations

Motivated Mocha

This delicious, creamy, mochalicious, energizing sugar-free elixir is full of protein, adaptogens, brain tonics, and medicinal herbs that promote heart health. While it supports the circulatory system, it floods our body with feel-good hormones such as serotonin and dopamine that have no sugar high or crash. Sometimes in the portal of the South, we call on our plant allies to help us bend the laws of time and space. This is the perfect elixir when we need a little extra push and power. I have used it to fuel myself with sustainable, joyful energy and creative productive flow when juggling the multiple roles and responsibilities in the Summer aspect of my life.

Yield: 1 serving

> ½ mug (120 ml) organic, fair-trade coffee
> ½ mug (120 ml) hemp mylk
> 2 tablespoon (10 g) cacao powder
> 1 tablespoon (7 g) collagen powder (or pea protein powder for vegetarians and vegans)
> 1 tablespoon (14 g) medicinal extracts of reishi, turkey tail, lion's mane mushrooms
> ¼ teaspoon (0.5 g) cinnamon powder
> ¼ teaspoon (0.5 g) macuna (dopamine bean)
> 1 teaspoon monk fruit (1.5 g) (zero-glycemic sweetener)
> 3 drops vanilla liquid stevia extract

1. Blend all ingredients on high until frothy. Serve and enjoy.

Lovers' Licking Chocolate

The climactic energies of summer nights, the moon in her luminous fullness, and the energies of creation in full expression may be enjoyed and enhanced in delicious ways with plants and lovers alike. This recipe is delicious, simple, and quick to prepare. It makes a delicious, thick, creamy chocolate ganache you can use to top a cake, drizzle over fresh strawberries and harden in the fridge, or lick off your lover's body on a full-moon night. It is full of healthy fats as well a mineral-rich and heart-healthy sacred cacao.

Yield: about 1¼ cups (300 ml)

> ½ cup (109 g) extra-virgin coconut oil
> ½ cup (162 g) maple syrup (Grade B if possible)
> ½ cup (43 g) cacao powder
> ½ teaspoon (2.5 ml) vanilla extract
> Pinch of Himalayan pink salt
> Generous dash (about ⅛ teaspoon, or 0.25 g) Ceylon cinnamon powder

1. Melt the coconut oil on low heat stirring and turning off once it is liquid. (On a hot summer day, your coconut oil may already be in liquid form.)

2. Mix in the maple syrup, cacao, and vanilla.

3. Finish with the salt and cinnamon.

4. Dip your fingers in and test the results.

Butterfly Blue Pea and Vanilla Chia-Seed Pudding

Chia seeds are a superfood loaded with nutrients, healthy fats, omega-3 fatty acids, fiber, antioxidants, and protein. They offer sustained energy, regulate blood sugar, improve digestion, and give us what our bodies need to move through the high-energy demands of the Summer portal. When infused in water, juice, or a nut mylk, they plump up, creating a tapioca-like texture. This can then be blended to make a mousse or served with fruit and sweetened for a delicious, healthy dessert. I love to get creative, and I make infinite variations of chia-seed puddings! Here is a beautiful creamy version that satisfies your sweet craving and is loaded with antioxidants and nutrition.

Yield: varies

1 cup (240 ml) butterfly blue pea infusion
2 tablespoons (38 g) coconut cream
½ teaspoon (2.5 ml) vanilla extract
⅛ cup (80 g) maple syrup or coconut sugar
¼ cup (44 g) chia seeds
Blueberries, strawberries, and raspberries

1. Blend the butterfly blue pea infusion with the coconut cream, the vanilla, and the sweetener of your choice.

2. For a mousse-like dessert, add the chia seeds and blend. For a tapioca-like consistency, pour the liquid into a jar and mix in the chia seeds.

3. Allow to sit for a few hours in the fridge, ideally overnight, stirring once if possible to prevent the seeds from clumping.

4. Cut the fruit into clear glass cups and alternate scooping layers of fruit and pudding on top. Serve with a drizzle of maple syrup (optional).

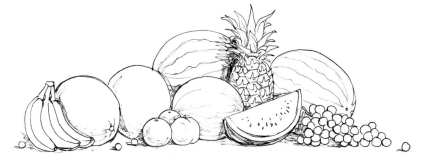

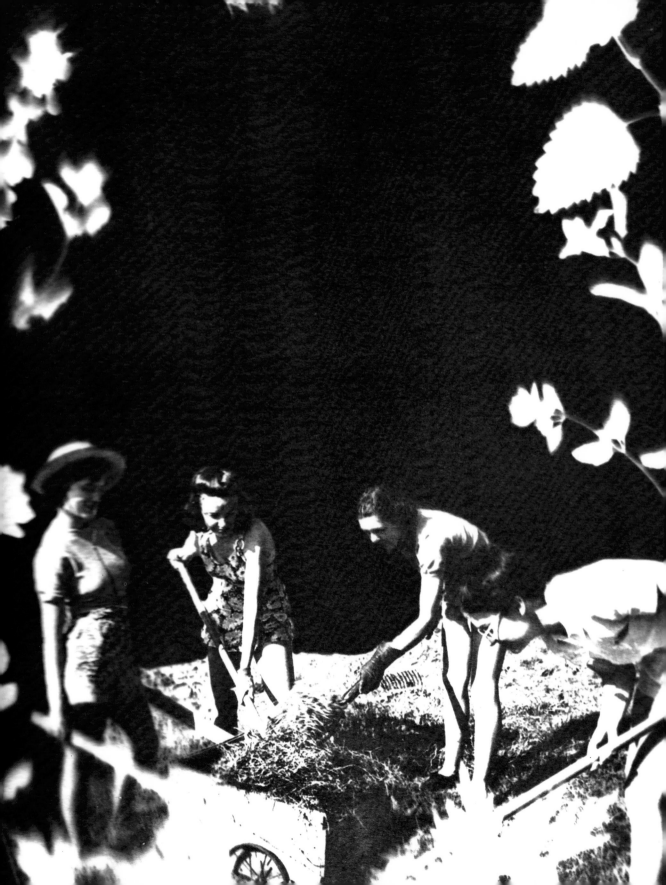

In the Garden, on the Earth

Summer is when the garden sings in glory. Fruits hang on trees, and every day there are fresh vegetables to harvest from the garden. Sometimes it feels like plants grow before our very eyes. Medicinal herbs flower and call out to pollinators and green witches, as many of them are ready for harvesting and medicine making.

The days are the longest of the year, and the energy of transformation is at its peak. This is the time to spend as much time as possible outside, in relationship with the gardens and lands you love. Think of the Mother archetype and how she lives in continual reciprocity with her children, community, and network of support and relations. This is the time to practice mothering land, to create healthy community, to spend time outside, and to socialize, expand your network, weave connections, and nourish reciprocal relationships. Now you generate bounty, learn directly from the plants that are in the peak of their expression, expand your abilities and apothecary, and transform yourself.

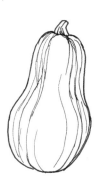
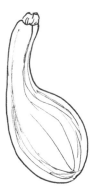

WHAT TO DO IN THE SUMMER

- Spend a lot of time with your garden, especially in the morning and evening.

- Observe, talk to, and listen to plants. They are in the peak of their expression.

- Trim plants back, harvest herbs to dry for tea and to make fresh medicine, tinctures, herbal vinegars, honeys, etc.

- Make a lot of medicine. The plants are abundant, the energies of transformation are high, and the days are long.

- Eat from the garden! The more you receive from the plants in gratitude, the more they grow and produce.

- Share your bounty, organize potlucks, eat outdoors, try new recipes, and eat local and fresh.

- Eat raw foods to stay cool.

- Stay hydrated.

- Compost and turn your compost pile when needed.

- Plant living mulch, such as the Summer cover crop buckwheat, or start planting cover crops for the Fall months.

- Feed your garden with compost and/or compost tea.

- Cover the soil with mulch or hay so it is not overexposed to the sun.

- Keep a garden journal. This is a time of learning, and we often forget what we intended to do differently or what worked really well.

- Share your bounty.

MAKING A GIFT POUCH

One of my sacred tools is a medicine pouch that I wear each time I teach, do ceremony, or need to call upon extra energy and assistance (such as going to court or having important meetings). I also give each of my apprentices a medicine pouch at the start of their apprenticeship and encourage them to carry little pinches of the plants they are working with near their hearts. All sorts of gifts from life and Nature have ended up in my medicine pouch—the body of a black widow spider that bit me, a piece of snakeskin I found, and more. Notice what appears to you and whether it symbolizes an energy you are working with.

A gift pouch is like a medicine pouch, but it carries offerings you collect for times of communion. It may contain meaningful gems, plants, and natural gifts. This pouch, too, builds in power and energy and is a beautiful tool to have—to share, in this portal of reciprocity.

Make your own pouch or find one made by an artisan. You can make a simple pouch by using a material that is meaningful to you or has your energy, such as an old dress or favorite shirt. Cut two U shapes about the size of your hand and sew them together, leaving the top open. Turn them inside out and tie the opening closed with a string. You can decorate it with beads and dip it into infusions of your plant allies in a ceremony of birthing your pouch into being. Begin a practice of collecting and making natural gifts as offerings and keep them in your pouch.

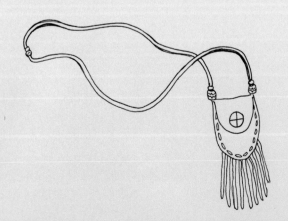

SUMMER RITUALS

In the season of Summer and the full moon portal, Witches draw on rituals of celebration to weave themselves into the climactic expression of energetic currents we have been encouraging since the darkness of Winter, through the awakening of Spring. Seeds that had been planted, prayers cast, visions in dark nights are now in ripe manifestation. While we never know what form our prayers will take, we pause in the Summer and give gratitude to the currents and mystery of life. We feed this portal with generosity, offerings, gratitude, devotion, and ceremonies of commitment.

The Summer Solstice is the holy day marking the highest point of solar expression, the longest day of the year, the peak of the masculine aspect of yang energy. In Europe, many villages celebrate by having a large bonfire, drinking and dancing into the night. Some make and burn male straw figures. While these are very pagan rituals, they have also been associated with celebrations of Saint John the Baptist Day, June 24 (just after the solstice). Some say the Christian church wove the strong pagan celebratory currents into Christian cosmology, moving the dates ever so slightly so the peak moment of the portal of magick was no longer accessed by the masses. In Poland, bonfires burn on Saint John's Day, and on the Summer Solstice maidens weave flower crowns, decorate them with candles, and offer them to flowing rivers.

Following are some of my most beloved Summer rituals that weave us into the generous, transformative portals of magick. All rituals of celebration, gratitude, community, and full-moon rituals and festivities weave us into the portals of the South.

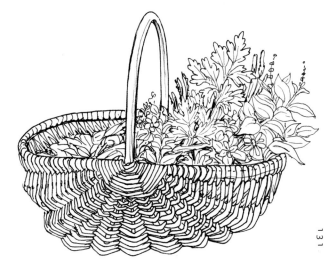

Ritual of Transformation:
Fire Ceremony

The portal of the South allows us to access the transformative power of the fire element. With fire, we can access instant release, activate our courage, fuel our prayers, and create meaningful change and miraculous transformation.

A Fire Ceremony can be simple or elaborate. For a more elaborate version, consider gathering with your coven or in a group of three Witches. This adds power to the ritual and the sacred container you create. It requires courage, which feeds the portals of transformation. Gather with the intention of releasing energies that do not serve your highest evolution and replace them with prayers for growth. Each Witch should bring her sacred tools, crystals, flowers or herbs that hold power for her. Together, create an altar and at the center place a vehicle of fire: a cauldron, a fire pit, or a candle. Create sacred space and cast a circle of protection for your ritual. Shift your consciousness with meditation, breathwork, tea, plant medicine, music—whatever helps you enter prayer space. Spend some time writing down in a piece of paper all that you are releasing. Write it in the affirmative: "On this day, I release . . ." Alternatively, come to the ritual already having written down all you are releasing in this ceremony. On another piece of paper, write what you are calling into the space that will be made.

Having called in the spirits and your guides, in sacred space, approach the fire one by one, breathe into your solar plexus, and speak out loud what you are releasing. This requires courage as you move radical truth from your body out through the sound of your unapologetic throat and the clarity of your third eye. When it is not your turn to speak, hold witness and ground the container in sacred space through your presence and prayers, assisting your sister or brother Witch in their release. Once you have spoken what you are releasing, burn the paper in the fire and affirm loudly, "And it is done!" The other witches repeat, affirming the spell, "And it is done!" Take a moment, breathing into your body, closing your eyes, and connecting to the space that has been made from what you have released. With your hands on your heart, speak what energies you are inviting into the space that has been made. It is good to keep it general but to be clear in your boundaries of what may enter this space within you. For example, you may call in trust in yourself, peace, faith, self-love, or the like.

A simpler version involves lighting a candle and burning paper with words you speak of what you release. When casting your circle and calling in the elements, always give gratitude to the spirits of fire and their miraculous ability to create transformation.

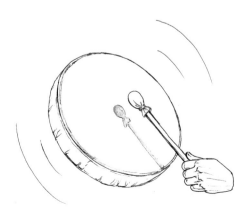

Marking Rites of Passage

The Summer portal corresponds to the Mother archetype, a time in our life when we are autonomous adults forging our own destiny, creating from a place of passion and purpose on a path of self-love, discovery, and self-expression. Entering this portal is often the first time we have the opportunity to create a rite of passage for ourselves, a practice we may then share with our children, friends, and family and draw on as we age. In the portal of transformation, we learn to fully digest our experiences in order to receive their medicine while also releasing old patterns or tendencies that hold us back from evolving into our next incarnation. A rite of passage allows us to mark the ending of an era and the birth of a new one. Rituals draw on the power of symbols and their associations in various levels of our consciousness. The embodied aspect of rituals that may seem theatrical from the outside allows us to engage all aspects of ourselves, including where experience and memory is stored: in the tissue, in our movements, words, songs, emotions, visions. When creating a ritual to mark a rite of passage, craft one that engages all senses. Grieve the end of one era in order to fully open to the gifts of the next.

Some examples of times when marking a rite of passage may be useful:

- Becoming a parent, marking the death of the maiden aspect

- Moving cities, communities, or countries

- Changing jobs

- Ending a relationship

- Release of a pregnancy through miscarriage or abortion

- Claiming a new title or a new role in your community, such as teacher or therapist

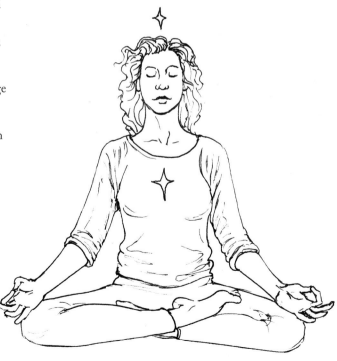

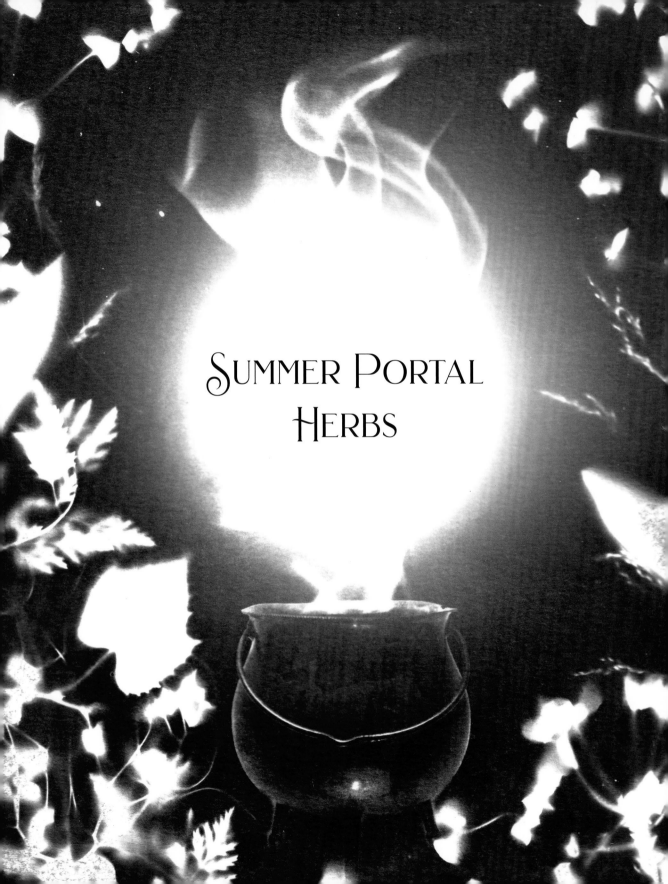

Summer Portal Herbs

plant profile

Cacao

LATIN NAME *Theobroma cacao*

FAMILY Malvaceae

Cacao is a seed, coming from an orange reddish fruit resembling a small papaya that grows directly off the trunk and branches of a tropical evergreen tree. Though cacao is native to Central America, most currently comes from Africa and Brazil. With a history of thousands of years as sacred medicine and "food of the gods," cacao continues to be a beloved plant consumed in large quantities by humans around the world, thus making it imperative we purchase certified fair-trade and organic cacao for ethical, environmental, and humanitarian reasons explained below.

HERBAL AND MEDICINAL PROPERTIES

- Nervous system stimulant: gives us energy and increases circulation
- Digestive: soothing to the stomach in bitter form
- Supportive to the heart: dilates blood vessels, lowers blood pressure
- Mineral rich
- Calming to the spirit, releases feelings of pleasure and joy

PLANT SPIRIT HEALING

I cannot imagine my life without cacao. It nourishes the root chakra, relaxes the parasympathetic nervous system, and brings feelings of ease, calm, and comfort. Cacao melts the body and heart into feelings of bliss, ranging from relaxation to feelings of giddy joy and euphoria. As an aphrodisiac and heart opener, cacao helps us connect lovingly to those around us. Boosting energy, motivation, joy, and mental clarity, cacao can fuel us in joyful creation and manifestation. As a plant spirit, she can be lover, seductress, or grandmother—her love is diverse and all encompassing. A dear friend and ethical chocolatière once pointed out that the guilt that some people feel when eating chocolate may be an energetic connection to sources that are unethical; indeed, some common candy brands use chocolate grown by slave children. How sad that an offering meant to elicit love can actually cause so much pain and suffering. For this reason, it is imperative that we boycott the big chocolate companies and purchase only fair-trade, organic cacao.

FAVORITE USES

- As food, making my own chocolate
- As drink and in elixirs
- As ceremonial drink, in meditation

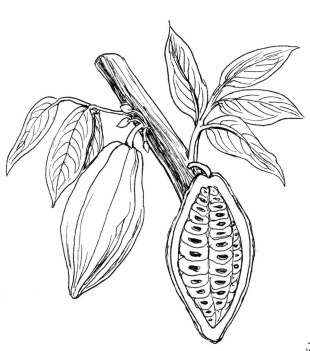

Schisandra

LATIN NAME *Schisandra chinensis*

FAMILY Schisandraceae

A perennial, deciduous climbing vine, schisandra grows in cool, temperate climates, having originated in northern China, Russia, and Korea. Harvest the red clusters of medicinal berries in the Fall for medicine—their seeds are shaped like kidneys. In traditional Chinese medicine, schisandra is called *wu wei zi*, the "five-taste berry"; it works on all meridians and organs and tonifies the three treasures: Qi, Jing, and Shen.

Those who are already frail or have a sensitive nervous system (classified as vata in Ayurvedic medicine) should use less schisandra, as she can be overstimulating to the nervous system and bring feelings associated with anxiety. For such individuals, I suggest adding a few berries to an infusion of oat straw.

HERBAL AND MEDICINAL PROPERTIES

- Adaptogen and longevity herb: used since ancient times as a plant for vigor, longevity, stamina, strength, and vigor
- Works on all systems of the body and all organs: strengthening to the immune system, nervous system, endocrine system, digestive system, cardiovascular system, and respiratory system (call her the miracle berry!)
- Nerve and mind tonic: energizing and stimulating, bringing mental clarity, focus, and motivation and uplifting with a brightening, antidepressant quality; amazing ally for chronic fatigue and stress; opening to the third eye and upper chakras
- Restorative to adrenals and kidneys: lifts us up out of darkness and lethargy, giving us energy while replenishing the adrenals and cleansing and tonifying the kidneys and liver

- Anti-inflammatory, antioxidant-rich beauty herb, with astringent properties that tonify the reproductive system and balance the water element in the body, making us more "juicy"
- Inspires creativity
- Aphrodisiac: a sexual tonic for both men and women that boosts libido, stamina, and zest for life
- Cleansing to the body: protective to the liver, boosts metabolism
- Heart tonic: supports circulation and integrity of blood vessels, balances blood sugar and cholesterol
- Immunomodulating: great for those with allergies and overactive immune systems as well as those who need a deep immune-system tonic, cancer-fighting ally, or support for chronic viral conditions such as HIV

PLANT SPIRIT HEALING

Schisandra is a superhero, a miracle berry of light, bright joy and zesty, juicy encouragement. She is one of my most beloved allies and has saved my life many times in moments of supreme challenge, darkness, and oppression. When you first drink her, the bright, lemony taste feels energizing, and the pucker of sour shows us how she tightens and tonifies mucous membranes, helping us contain and move our water, creativity, energy, and vitality in a vessel of integrity. Balancing to all chakras, she increases chi, cleans out toxins, moves stagnant emotional and physical energy, and brightens and clears the energetic body, mind, spirit and heart. I often feel her spirit cleaning the windshield of my third eye, bringing clarity and focus to my visions while offering a sassy, supportive, sisterly "You got this!" I have created some real miracles in my life thanks to her support and uplifting energy. She has motivated me, inspired me, and gotten me unstuck in times of great hardship. If you work with her consistently for a month, you will see significant changes in your energy, and you may also begin to embody some of her sassy personality. She is not shy, she knows what she loves, and goes for it with confident joy and self-love!

FAVORITE USES

- Hot overnight infusion, enjoyed cold the following day (drink daily for a month)
- Mixed with oat straw for a more calming version
- Mixed with butterfly blue pea or hibiscus, as in recipes
- As a base for fabulous medicinal summertime cocktails with vodka and soda water

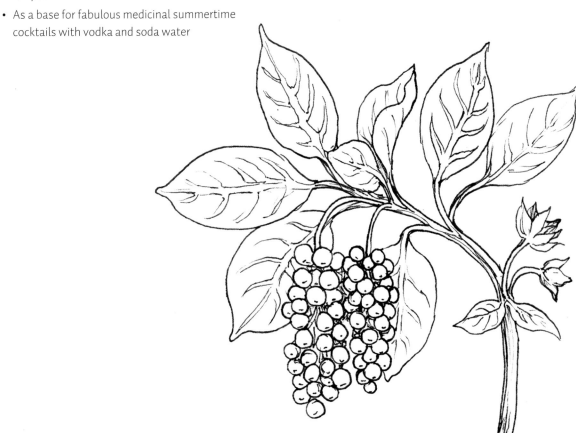

plant profile

Mint

LATIN NAME *Mentha* spp.

FAMILY Lamiaceae (mint family)

Low-growing, widely spreading, hardy perennial herbs native to Eurasia, North America, southern Africa, and Australia, mints are widely distributed throughout the temperate areas of the world and have naturalized in many places. These plants have a square stem and bright leaves that are harvested in the Spring and Summer and cut back after they have gone to flower and seed.

HERBAL AND MEDICINAL PROPERTIES

- Carminative and aromatic: wonderful after a meal to help digest and soothe the belly, especially in cases of gas, bloating, lethargy, and overeating
- Antispasmodic: relaxing to muscles, helpful for cramps and menstrual flow
- Diaphoretic: increases circulation and lowers body temperature
- Decongestant: opening to breath, lungs, and nasal passages
- Calming to the nervous system
- Supports mental clarity, focus, and clear communication
- Antimicrobial and anti-inflammatory

PLANT SPIRIT HEALING

Peppermint and spearmint bring us to the joyful, sunny garden where the Earth is moist and the body feels grounded and revitalized. Nourishing, energizing, and grounding, this plant spirit is an ally for moving stuck energy, bringing vitality and light, and purifying our vibration. The mints move energy in the sacral chakra and solar plexus and can be activating, gently uplifting, and encouraging. The current of vital Earth energy continues to move up the chakras to a heart that opens with an expanding breath and greater clarity and perspective in the mind. The air element in mints has a strong presence and opens the centers of communication and the upper chakras. These plants have a confident, joyful disposition, helping us connect to the feelings of what it means to thrive, woven deeply into all the elements and the fabric of the nourished Earth.

FAVORITE USES

- In herbal formulas to improve taste and increase circulation
- In fresh herbal juices
- As an after-dinner digestive following heavy meals
- One of the best herbs to relieve gas
- Pairs incredibly well with watermelon (see recipes)
- In food medicine: I love to make a quinoa tabbouleh with generous amounts of parsley and mint.

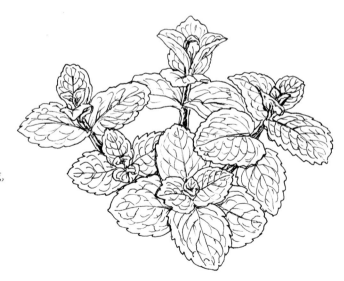

Calendula

LATIN NAME *Calendula officinalis*

FAMILY Asteraceae/Compositae (aster family)

This flowering annual reseeds itself easily, creating beautiful, daisy-like, velvet-smooth flowers, consisting of concentric rows of ray florets, colors ranging from yellow to orange, growing to about a foot. Calendula (pot marigold) is native to southern Europe but has spread, growing in temperate regions around the world. Incredibly easy to propagate, the seeds resemble lions' jaws, and the flower resembles the sun.

HERBAL AND MEDICINAL PROPERTIES

- Vulnerary: wound healer, topically in salves, oils, teas, and washes; internally soothing, healing, and anti-inflammatory as well
- Antimicrobial, antiviral, immunostimulant
- Antispasmodic: relaxing to tension in the body, an ally supportive of menstrual flow and a magickal herb for the womb and sacral chakra
- Lymphatic: moves the waters in the body and cleanses the lymphatic system
- Calendula has ancient associations with goddesses of many cultures such as Xochiquetzal, the Aztec love goddess; Mother Mary (source of the name marigold); the Indian Goddess Mahadevi; the Greco-Roman Diana and Apollo; and many more
- There is much lore and magick associated with protection spells, love spells, and secret teachings of life and death.

PLANT SPIRIT HEALING

While her simple beauty can easily be overlooked, behind the childlike joy is deep magick and portals that open gateways to the mysteries. I have received profound teachings and healing from the marigold, including instant healing with herbal bathing associated with problems I was experiencing in my womb. She bridges the lands of the living and the dead, the masculine and feminine aspects, light and dark. In meditation, she calms the spirit, soothes and nourishes the water element and brings gentle inspiration, movement, and creative flow. Opening to the heart chakra and gently consciousness shifting, I find this plant spirit very accessible and available as a healer and guide.

FAVORITE USES

- Edible flower on salads
- For salves, oils, and other beauty uses, including baby bum-rash balm
- Flower essences
- In gardening, for pollinators, as an easy, beautiful herb and groundcover
- For tea, tincture, infused honey, and infused vinegar
- For bath and shamanic meditations—an incredible teacher plant

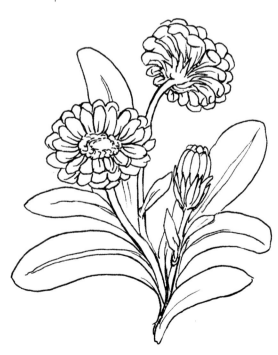

plant profile

Hibiscus

LATIN NAME: *Hibiscus rosa, Hibiscus sabdariffa*

LATIN NAME Hibiscus sabdariffa

FAMILY Malvaceae (Mallow Family)

Hibiscus is an evergreen shrub with flossy, oval deep-green leaves and large, beautiful, fully open five-petaled flowers ranging from pink to red, with her reproductive parts sticking out on a long filament. Native to North Africa and Southeast Asia, she grows in tropical regions around the world.

HERBAL AND MEDICINAL PROPERTIES

- Astringent, cooling herb: used often in tropical folk medicine to cool the body, cleanse the urinary-tract system, relieve fevers, and tonify the reproductive organs
- Anti-inflammatory and antihypertensive: lowers blood pressure and is rich in antioxidants, vitamin C, and nutrients.
- Antiparasitic and antibacterial: a great ally for urinary-tract and bladder infections
- Aphrodisiac: heart chakra opener with ancient magickal lore connected to the Goddess

PLANT SPIRIT HEALING

Beautiful hibiscus embodies a sensual, creative, feminine, and loving energy, supporting us in dissolving sexual trauma, cleansing and purifying the womb space, and bringing the spirit of her ever-renewing blossoms. She teaches self-love and treating oneself as sacred. A great ally for healthy boundaries, she opens the heart and has helped many women reconnect to their sexuality, sensuality, and innocence. Cooling and hydrating in the summer months, she replenishes us and makes us feel like a goddess.

FAVORITE USES

- Hibiscus glycerite
- Iced tea (see recipes, pages 124 to 125)
- Edible leaves in salads
- Flower essence

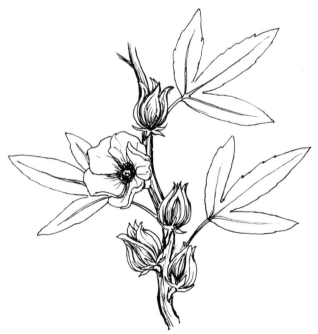

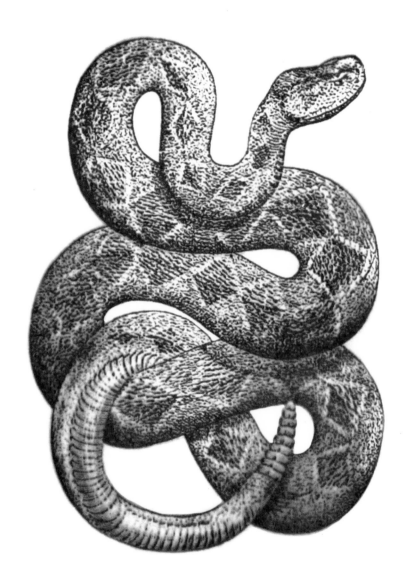

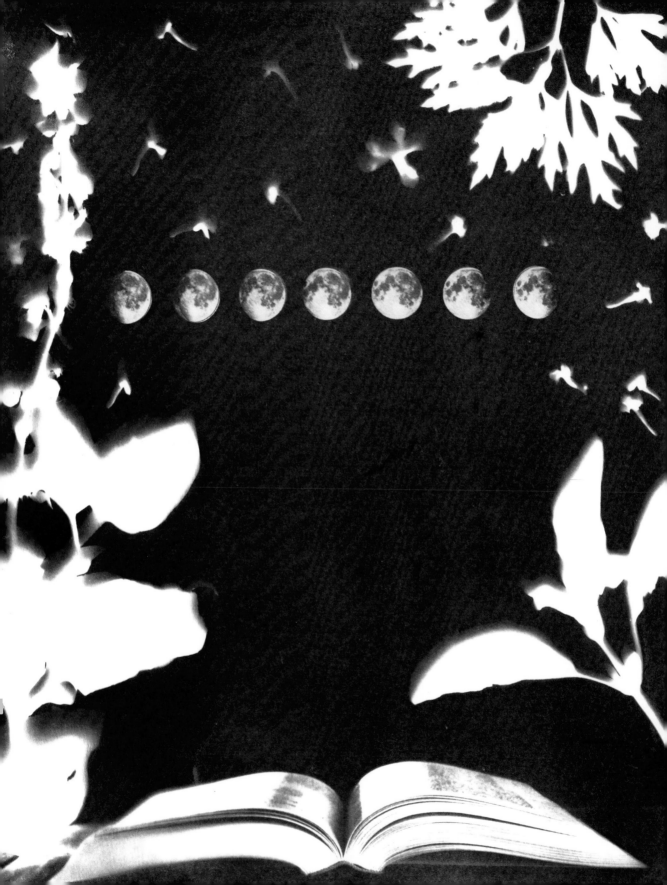

South Portal Journal Prompts

Reflect on the element of fire in you. These are some examples.

Fire element in balance

- Healthy sense of self, self-motivation, being fueled by a zest for life, ability to follow through, act, and create in a consistent, effective way (balanced with earth)

- Passion, purpose, playfulness, joy, optimism, warm disposition (balanced with earth, water, and air)

- Good boundaries, but not rigid (balanced with earth, water, and air)

- Ability to take risks, step outside of the status quo, and confront injustice

Fire element out of balance

- Jealousy, being quick to anger, bad temper, volatility (needs grounding of earth and cooling and calming of water)

- Inflammation in the body, rashes, eczema, dry skin (needs demulcent, hydrating, anti-inflammatory herbs)

- Really quick metabolism, does not assimilate nutrients (needs more earth and water, grounding foods high in fats and healthy grains and veggies, and consistent, earth-paced eating habits)

- Unmotivated, depressed, lethargic (needs more fire to balance earth)

Reflect on how you can cultivate balance in a time and culture that pushes doing and giving.

- Which practices of the North portal help balance the energies of the South for you?

- How can you mother yourself? What are your deepest emotional needs right now, and how can you support yourself in receiving what is most nourishing for your soul?

- Make a list of all the things in our life and plans that feel like a big, resounding *yes*!

- Make a list of all the things, people, and plans in your life that feel like a "meh" or a no.

- What do you most want to transform right now? In yourself? In your life? In your community? In the world?

- Find inspiration in an activist or one of your heroes. How did or do they live their life in courage?

- What achievements can you celebrate right now? Make a long list! Remember all the things that you have started as seeds and hopes. Take the time and do a ritual of celebration honoring all that you have accomplished, all the ways you have grown. The full moon is an optimal time for this ritual.

- Create a ritual marking a transformation in your life. Perhaps you have literally become a mother. How could you ritualize the death of the Maiden, or the new beginnings that await you? Perhaps you are turning fifty this year. How can you deeply honor the significance of the transformations in your life?

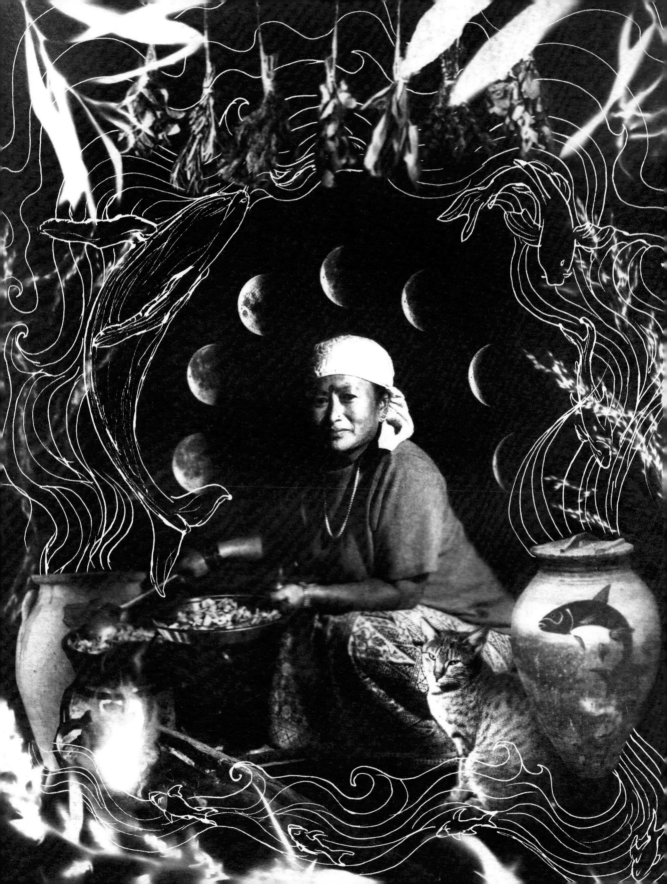

Chapter 6

EARTH MAGICK & MEDICINE OF FALL

Harvest & Compost: Wisdom & Magick | West · Water · The Wise Woman

---

The Portal of the West at a Glance

ELEMENT Water

TIME OF DAY Sunset | 4:00–10:00 p.m.

MOON PHASE Waning

SEASON OF SOLAR YEAR Fall | September, October, November

EARTH HOLY DAYS Mabon (Fall Equinox) | September 21–24; Samhain (Halloween), All Saints' Day, and Day of the Dead | October 31–November 2

WHEEL OF LIFE ARCHETYPE Wise Woman | Age 42–63

ENERGIES Waning, wisdom and discernment, harvesting, gratitude, retreating, rest, going inward, release, grief, intimacy, compassion, mysteries, dreaming, cleansing, divination, intuition, healing, magick and shamanism

HEALING HERBS

Adaptogens & Deep immune tonics Astragalus, Siberian ginseng, ashwagandha, shatavari, rhodiola

Surface immune stimulants to ward off colds Echinacea, elderflower and berry, ginger, garlic, olive leaf, yerba santa

Medicinal mushrooms Shiitake, maitake, turkey tail, reishi (please do not use Chaga as it is overharvested)

Nourishing roots Burdock, dandelion, marshmallow, turmeric

Nervines Skullcap, passionflower, linden, blue vervain, kava kava, peach leaf, damiana

Heart openers Rose, kava kava, linden, peach leaf, jasmine, motherwort, tulsi

Dream magick and consciousness Shifters Blue lotus, kava kava, mugwort, passionflower, damiana

TENDING THE GARDEN Harvesting; cutting back dead brush; composting; clearing away, putting gardens to rest for winter; planting cover crops

APOTHECARY Harvesting medicinal plants for drying or tinctures; digging up medicinal roots; tincturing; canning; fire cider and immune vinegars; making immune-boosting medicine; ritual baths; dream medicine

RITUALS Rituals of release, grief work, shamanic journeying, dream magick, herbal bathing, flower waters, cord cutting, midwifing death

Gaia Speaks

Beloved one.
You are wild, yet you are wise.
You expand, yet you are contained.
You are both the vessel and the sacred healing waters.

Gone are the days of spilling your nectars.
The children that drank from your breasts have grown and flown,
your nest is now your own,
your blood returning to your cup for you alone to hold.

Reflect on the journeys of your days
and know you can travel anywhere in your dreams and soul.
No thing is your boundary and
never before were your boundaries so honoring
to the integrity of your Self.

Take your drum in hand and rattle.
Stomp your bones deeper into the Earthen floor.
Sour your spirit with the winged ones
and the waning moon that calls you deeper.

You are medicine woman.
Like cured fruit your sweetness is deep in your leathered skin.
You have sprouted life and midwifed death.
You learned to sit with pain and keep the company of broken hearts.
You are not afraid and so
you are free.
You know.
You see.
You re-member.

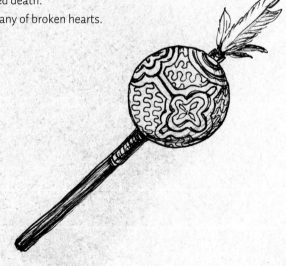

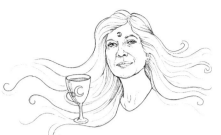

Release to Regenerate Yourself, Wise Witch

Fall Equinox. A moment of perfect balance. We hang suspended with the light of day equal to the length of night. Behind us are the long days of Summer—the full gardens, ripe with fruit of our labor, and fields of grain. The days then were full and hot, and all of Nature pushed us to expand, work, and produce abundantly so that now, in the season of fall, in the middle years of our life, we can reap a harvest from all we have sown.

Ahead of us are the waning days, the darkening nights with mists that cover mountains like a blanket, mornings that smell like composting leaves exhaling sighs of release into the Earth. Like those who came before us, we celebrate the harvests and give gratitude for all we have, acknowledging our efforts of the season past. We prepare for the deep dream of Winter by canning tomatoes, filling the cellars, storing the grain for the cold months ahead, when the Earth will dream under blankets of snow.

Now is the time of the Wise Woman—she who practices discernment and uses her energy wisely. The energy of Gaia is waning. The Sun King goes into the underworld on the Fall Equinox to be reborn on the Winter Solstice. This is the time to release. We put down the heavy baskets of Summer responsibilities, obligations, and too many yeses. We make ourselves lighter so we can move into nonlinear realms, into dreamtime, into the deep watery places in our bodies that feel the mysteries, so we can flow on the river that will take us to the void of Winter's renewal.

In the garden, we cut back dead brush. The plants have pulled their vital energy into their roots as they prepare to dream in the dark soil of the Winter Earth. The parts

that had extended toward the sun appear dead. We cut these brown branches, twigs, and grasses back, feeling the things in our lives we are ready to release. With some of these twigs, we make kindling bundles to start Winter fires; all that has died is feeding new life to come. And so we reflect on what we can give death to, in order to create more life when the time is ripe. Fall is a good time for cord-cutting ceremonies, rituals of release, and practices of discernment, forgiveness, and compassion.

The West's portals of release open to you each day at dusk, each waning moon, each Fall season, and in the middle years of your life. Use this time wisely to put down your baskets of doings and overcommitments. Cut away your overextended ways that spread you thin and far, and draw yourself back into your wholeness. Take your whole and holy Self and dive into the West to be carried on the rivers of the Great Mystery, dissolving into the oceanic fertile void of the North. From this darkness of the Winter's night, like a crescent new moon, you will emerge renewed, blossoming in unimaginable Spring miracles and ripening into Summer fullness as the garden of You.

Release to regenerate yourself,
Wise Witch.

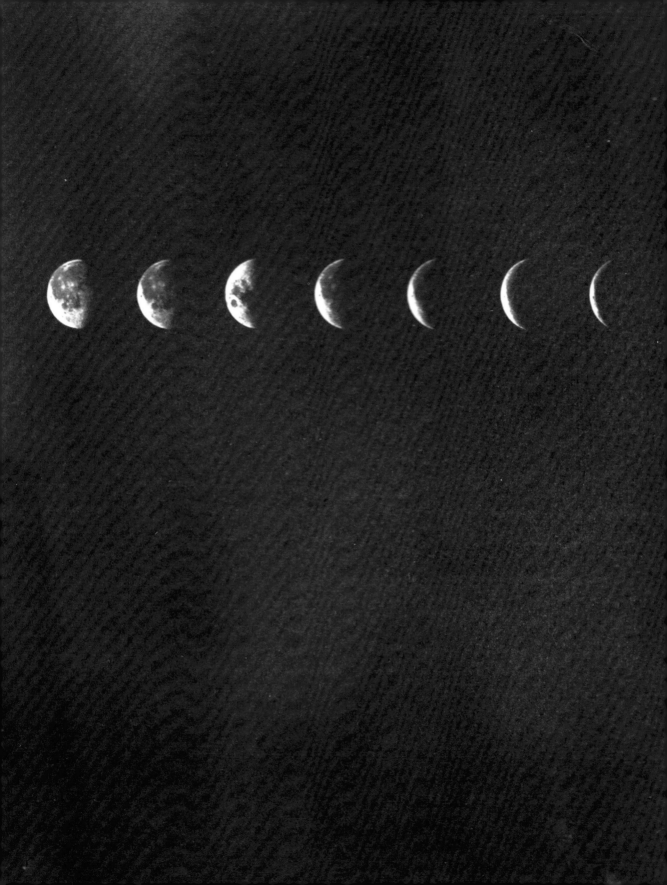

Entering the Portals of the West

The portal of the West is the time of waning energy present in all of Nature's cycles. In the twenty-four-hour cycle, we enter this portal by guiding ourselves away from the active part of the day and slipping into the sunset waters of a healing evening to prepare for the deep, restorative rest of the night. The West portal also opens us to the mysteries of the waning moon, when blankets of starlit black skies slip over our luminous fullness, cradling us to darkness so we may be reborn with a new moon. In the solar year, the season of Fall carries us towards the end of the Gregorian calendar, spanning the months of September, October, and November in the northern hemisphere, with the Fall Equinox (September 21–24) marking the official start of the year's final exhale. In the wheel of our lives, the West corresponds to our middle-age years and the archetype of the Wise Woman.

In our herbal garden, medicinal roots are ready for harvest. With the aerial parts of the plants dying back, the roots hold stronger medicine, more chi. We dig up the echinacea, burdock, and yellow dock roots. With dirt beneath our nails and the smell of the damp Earth exhaling as we dig our medicine, our root chakra receives nourishment. Our energetic body drops into the pace of the Earth, grounding down. Our airy minds quiet, the nervous system calms. This is the time to work with the plants that release tension in the mind and body. Many of us get tightly wound over the busy Summer months; some of us burn out. Now is the time to slow down, go deeper, release, and let go.

Our apothecary grows in this time of release. The Earth transfers her abundance to the Witch, who alchemizes the gifts of Nature and makes medicine. The roots may be tinctured, seeds collected for Spring. It is time to make immunity syrups and medicines to protect us in the colder months when viruses and flus run rampant. Elderberry syrups, echinacea tinctures, burdock bone broths, and fire cider are some of my favorite Fall recipes. Dream elixirs, herbal baths, and smoke blends shift our consciousness into the watery realms of the West, quieting the busy mind and awakening our intuition.

In all wheels great and small, this is the time to shift our energy inward, harvesting the fruits of our solar labors in gratitude and preparing for the darker times to come.

Entering the West Each Evening

In the wheel of the day, West corresponds to the late afternoon and evening, roughly from 4:00 to 10:00 p.m. To ride the regenerative currents of the wheels, enter the early afternoon by transitioning your activities and energy away from the daytime solar/yang/masculine energy of expansion and doing and toward a more yin/feminine/healing energy of relaxation and nourishment.

Sometimes it is challenging to shift gears from doing to being. The small wheel of each day allows us to practice this unwinding every evening. Because learning to live regeneratively often involves remembering ancient ways not taught or promoted by modern culture, we are lucky to have the medicinal plants and the power of rituals to help us create new habits and retrain our nervous system. The more we practice each evening with plants and rituals of release and relaxation, the better we become at riding the currents of the West each lunar month, each Fall, ultimately becoming wiser and more powerful in our middle age.

The meal of the West is dinner, which in many homes is when all members of the family come together after an expansive and busy day. They connect around the "hearth" and heart of the home, give gratitude, and share a nourishing meal. As Witches, we use the power of conscious intention to guide ourselves and our loved ones into deeper levels of connection, healing, and love. The simple act of sharing dinner can become deeply healing and nourishing or, if eaten when stressed or rushed, can lead to indigestion, loss of energy, and weight gain. Make dinnertime sacred. Being present with one another feeds the heart and our need for intimate connection. If dining alone, make an extra effort to show your spirit that you know how to court yourself. Use food vessels you find beautiful, and bless your food. Eating slowly, gratefully, and mindfully promotes good digestion and helps us stay at our natural weight.

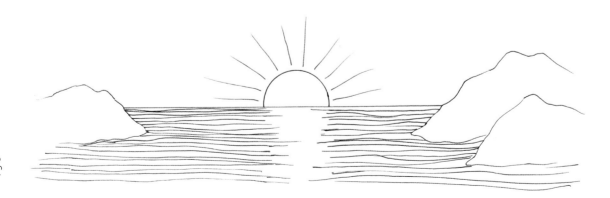

Evening Practices to Weave You into the West

These are good practices for the "Fall" portion of the day, the lunar cycle, the year, and your life.

- Drink nervine tea or Kava Bliss Elixir (see page 161) to transition from the workday to the evening.

- Cook a nourishing meal.

- Slow down, relax, and rest.

- Give yourself a massage.

- Spend some time in a ritual bath, sauna, bath, hot tub, or any other water.

- Take an evening stroll alone or with a loved one.

- Watch the sunset.

- Spend time with Nature's water—walk on the beach or take a swim in wild water

- Create a sensual, nourishing home environment that holds you sweetly.

- Say no to anything that feels draining. Cancel social engagements that feel like an effort.

- End your workday.

- Read poetry, listen to music or storytelling, play an instrument, or do some crafting.

- Make medicine

- Meditate, pray, do some shamanic journeying, or do some healing work.

- Give gratitude for your day, reflect on your day, or journal.

- Help a friend, share a meal, and build safe and loving communities and relationships.

- Give yourself a little alone time, even if only for ten minutes.

- Cuddle with your pet, kids, or loved one—or with yourself.

RELEASING WITH THE WANING MOON

The waning moon of the West portal is a roughly eight- to ten-day period each month following the full-moon portal of South and bringing us into the new-moon portal of North.

We humans are deeply woven into the cycles of the moon, as may be seen in our most ancient and modern rituals and religions, in diverse cultural customs, in our art and music, in our farming, and in our biology and reproductive cycle. The biological bond between humans and the moon is also incredibly powerful and visible in a woman's body and menstrual cycle, which follows the phases of the moon, shifting from twenty-eight to thirty days. Women often bleed on the full or new moon, and then ovulate on the opposite side of the wheel. When women live together, their menstrual cycles often align, and they may begin bleeding at the same time. The womb is a body of water. Like the ocean, its tides and flow are influenced by the cycles of the moon.

When using the moon to chart your fertility and menstrual cycle, use the Wheel of the Year (see page 7). Mark your first day of bleeding as the dark moon, regardless of the moon's actual phase in the sky. The cycle of the waning moon occurs after ovulation, which corresponds to the full moon. If a woman's egg has not been fertilized, she may experience a drop in hormones that feels like a descent in energy, or even sadness or grief. When we follow the regenerative moon cycle, we support our bodies with nourishing herbal medicines at this time. As we approach the new moon and time to bleed, we can call on plants such as mugwort or angelica that assist us in the shedding of our uterine wall and the release of our moon blood.

The "waning moon" phase is the Fall of the reproductive cycle. the time for her to prepare for the Winter of bleeding time. To ride the regenerative currents of renewal with the menses, a woman should rest when she bleeds and stay warm and nourished with nourishing broths. The Fall is a time to prepare nourishing foods, cancel appointments, and find babysitters. Then, in the Spring of the woman's reproductive cycle, she feels revived and renewed.

In the creative cycle of business and who we are in the world, the waning moon is a good time for accounting, reflecting on the month, gathering lessons learned, finishing projects, and planning for some rest and downtime.

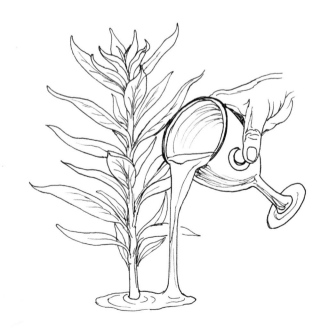

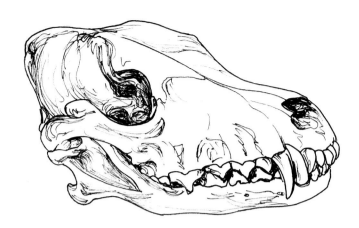

Midwifing Death in the Fall

By now, we understand how to embody the waning energies of the West. Nature offers the deeper teachings of letting go, releasing, composting, and midwifing death in order to create more life in moons to come. It is in the garden that we can heal our relationship to death and learn how to tend to it in order to create life. Without death, there is no life. The garden where seeds effortlessly sprout and life blossoms in ecstasy is also the one rich in death and decay. Without compost, without an ecosystem digesting that which is allowed to return to the Earth, there can be no food for new life to come.

In our modern culture, growth, expansion, life, and eternal youth and beauty are prized and exalted. Meanwhile, we often don't know how to approach death, much less midwife and walk with hand in hand it. When we do not allow for the season of Fall to enter our relationships, creative projects, bodies, minds, and souls, we overextend Summer, trying to do, produce, and expand—and we burn out. Being unable to tend to death in our lives also prevents us from rebirthing ourselves, and we may become stuck, weak, uninspired, depressed, or ill.

If we follow the currents of Nature, we have the opportunity to accept and love her dormant state. After all, it can remind us that we too can be dormant and ugly, that we do not always have to reveal ourselves as beautiful for all to enjoy. What is invisible is life-giving and most important in the dark times of the year. Furthermore, when allowed to descend into the fertile darkness of the soil, we enter the currents of regeneration that lead to a magical moment in new growth of the Spring.

Nature is not afraid of death. Death is a sweet return into the wholeness from which new life emerges.

The Wise Woman Archetype

In the wheel of our lifetime, we enter the Wise Woman stage in middle age, from roughly age forty-two to sixty-three These are the wisdom years that, when tended to with intention, allow us to become sages and the kind of elders that can guide an entire culture into wholeness and balance. We arrive in the ripeness of our middle years following the Summer fruiting of our life, which is associated with the Mother archetype, the element of Fire, and the direction of South.

Working with archetypes allows us to connect to universal energies, offering the most potent medicine when we move beyond the literal, into the formless. Thus, these archetypes are available to people of any gender, any age, with or without children, and so on. One of the primary energetic differences between our Summer/Mother phase and our Fall/Wise Woman phase is how we move our life-force energy from our creative center (sacral chakra) and how this energy creates form and ripples into the formless. Also, there is a shift in how we take in information through our third eye, how we cast visions into the world, and the relationship between the third eye center and our solar plexus, the center of will and action.

At the end of our personal Summer, sweaty, sun-kissed, enlivened, and a little tired, we sit down in the late afternoon of our lives, "the magick hour," look around, and appreciate the beauty of creation. We begin the process of shifting our energy, slowing down, and ripening the fruit of our labor. In our Fall, we plant fewer seeds and tend to the trees that are already mature and established. There is work there too, and it is the season of gathering the fruits of our labor, sharing our bounty, and preserving our richness to carry us through the Winter of our lives.

With abundance in the very late Summer and Fall of our lives, we gather with our loved ones for celebrations of the harvest. We also have good boundaries and are wise enough not to become entangled in other people's confusion. We move through relationships and decisions with greater discernment, perspective, and experience. We learn how to allow life to unfold, honoring the place of the Great Mystery and moving away from forcing life in accordance with our vision of how things should be and our strong, fiery will. As we no longer push ourselves, others, or life as the primary way to manifest form and projects, we can settle into a deeper trust in the flow and timing of life.

Like the balance of light and dark at the Fall Equinox, we also have a healthy balance of cultivating our inner and outer life. We are often still engaged in our community, while also desiring more time alone for reflection or to feed our spiritual well, which inspires how we express our being in the world. The element of water in the West reveals a greater ability to hold and move a variety of emotions without being washed away and losing ourselves. Intuition and psychic abilities grow as does our spiritual practice. We do shamanic journeys and dream work, or spend more time in the nonlinear realms. The "right brain" tends to be rewarding and deeply nutritive to the soul.

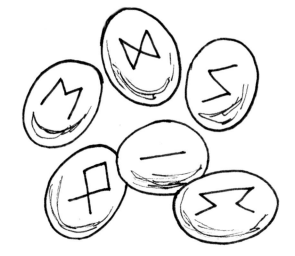

For women, the time of birthing children wanes with changing hormones as we enter menopause. In many cultures, the time when a woman stops bleeding is associated with greater spiritual power. The life-giving energy in the form of blood we offer to the Earth each month in our Mother phase is considered to now shift inward, the energy remaining for the woman alone.

For men, sexual hormones also change. Testosterone tends to diminish, corresponding to the waning solar aspect of their sexuality. Middle-aged men tend to become more sensitive, entering the waters of the West and often coming into deeper relationship with their emotions, intuition, dreams, and sensitivities.

People in the Fall of their lives have a breadth of life experience behind them. As we know ourselves more and appreciate the gift and impermanence of life more, we often begin to prioritize the rituals and self-care that allow us to feel well, vital, and balanced. There are many people who begin a journey of health in their middle years, remarking that they now feel better than they did in their twenties. The Wise one uses herbs, rituals, exercise, and self-care for both increasing energy and vitality and to bring her into deeper states of relaxation and restorative healing.

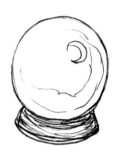

HEALING THE WISE WOMAN WITHIN

Some people arrive at this portal with empty baskets and fear in their minds. Those who lack courage in the portal of the South may have held themselves back, never fully committing to a project or seeing it through. Sometimes childhood trauma causes a part of our spirit to stay stuck in the Spring until the wound can be healed and transformed. Being stuck in the Maiden archetype of Spring may involve fearing growing up and taking responsibility. Or it could involve always seeking new experiences and adventures, moving energy in a scattered way, and never fully tending a project into fruition. Others do commit themselves fully into a creation only to find that life and the Great Mystery have brought blight through, and the gardens they've tended for years have been unexpectedly destroyed, leaving them brokenhearted and confused. They find their baskets empty at the time of harvest in the West.

Those arriving without much bounty in their middle years may experience fear, doubt, or a spiritual crisis. This is where Witches draw on our ability to bend time and space. We work within the gateways that open in each portal to create miracles and regenerate our lives. Even if the arc of your life has led to an impoverished garden, the portals of the South will forever open to you, inviting you to meet each day with courage and action, to raise the energies of manifestation at each full moon, and to ride the solar strength of the long days of summer, working hard and dedicating yourself to your new, inspired creations and commitments.

The days of Fall may not be as long and energetic as those of the previous season, but the Wise Woman who has worked hard in the Summer now knows how to work wiser. She is discerning with the use of her energy, a maturity within that lends itself to a beautiful ripening, deepening, and maturation of her creations and projects. She no longer says yes to every project, social invitation, work commitment, or child. The Wise Woman pauses. She knows there is no rush to reply. By first checking in with her truth, she can cut chaos out of her life. You will often hear a Wise Woman answering, "Hmm, let me think about it" or, "I'll get

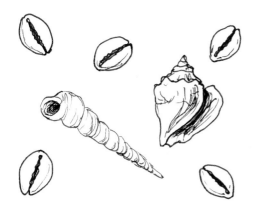

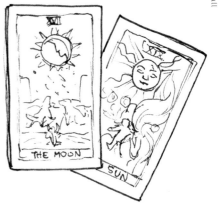

back to you." The Wise Woman is clear with her yeses and her nos. She can create much magick, abundance, and magnificence in her life in a way that is often much more her own, in accordance with her strengths, truths, and talents and with a greater honoring of self-care, rest, and pleasure. Practicing discernment and listening to the deep yes and no from within helps heal and strengthen the vessel of the Wise Woman, sealing any energetic leaks, and cultivating power and trust in Self.

Indeed, there is no harsh line separating the South from the West. Each of us finds the climax of our energetic output to vary, waxing and waning with each day, month, and year. These days, many people have families later than we used to or start business in their golden years. Again, our age does not matter as much as how we use our energy. You may also find yourself professionally in your Wise Woman stage while just entering life as a new mother or a new relationship that expands your mind like the springtime of the maiden. By entering the portals on the wheel available each day, month, and year with intention, even a young maiden can begin developing and drawing on the gifts of her inner sage.

We are Witches. We are timeless.

EARTH MEDICINE OF THE WEST: CONSCIOUSNESS-SHIFTING PLANTS

Plants are our elders. Humans came to be on the planet thanks to the plant life that moved from ocean to land and created oxygen. Many of our medicinal herbs have been on this planet longer than humans. They have adapted over thousands of years to diverse ecosystems, climates, and conditions. They carry with them resilience that becomes medicine for our human bodies, strengthening us and making us more adaptable. They also carry their signature, spirit, and blend of elements—just as each of us does. Plants have consciousness and personality, and they open portals in our minds, emotional bodies, and spirits, providing an embodied experience of a state of consciousness that may be different than how we are used to experiencing ourselves.

The plants of the West are often grounding and slowing to the nervous system, opening to the heart and sacral chakra, nourishing to the element of water inside of us, and activating to our dreaming, intuitive mind. They give us an embodied experience of relaxation, bringing us into the deeper brain waves where we can heal our nervous systems, retrain our minds, and come to experience ourselves as relaxed, anxiety free, and more creative—sometimes for the first time in our lives.

Many people these days struggle with chronic stress, anxiety, and overactive minds. If this becomes your norm, you may begin to identify with your anxiety (or depression or other state of consciousness), creating a story that you are "simply an anxious person." Working with plant-spirit medicine allows us to shift and experience different states of consciousness. The relaxing plants of the West often cause people who have identified as anxious to suddenly realize, "Wow, in this moment, my breath, heart, and mind are actually calm and quiet. This feels good." With the new awareness that we are not our anxiety, or that we are capable of lying down and relaxing, we can use the power of our intention and awareness, along with the ancient healing gifts of the herbs, to compost old

and limiting stories about ourselves and become more expansive, self-loving, and wise.

Nervine herbal teas are perfect allies to help us enter this portal and transition into a more relaxed state. They guide us through the West as a time of transition, teaching us how to relax, release, and receive healing on both a physical and an emotional level. Nervines are herbs that relax and calm the nervous system, such as skullcap, motherwort, holy basil, lavender, and chamomile. Making a warm tea or elixir with these plants relieves anxiety, calms the thinking and analytical brain that has been dominating our workday, and gets us into the left brain, where we can be more creative and imaginative. Some nervines, such as kava kava, skullcap, and blue lotus, are also antispasmodic, which means they release tension, stress, cramps, and tightness from the body, giving us not only a calm mind but also a deeply relaxed, pain-free body.

Sedatives, herbs that are even stronger than nervines, can help us get the restorative sleep we need. Although deep, restorative sleep is associated with the portal of the North and the time of Winter, the West is our time of transition, which prepares us to enter that regenerative dark time. The pace of our modern culture

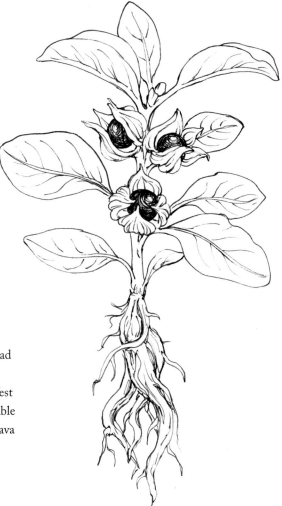

pushes us to prolong the workday, and the transition time of the West is often omitted—people go from work to passing out. Lengthening the active state, working late, and omitting the transition state can lead to insomnia, anxiety, sleep disorders, adrenal fatigue, depletion, and even depression. The portals of the West and North, the times of darkness, aren't seen as valuable in our modern culture. Sedatives, such as hops and kava kava in high doses, help us stop resisting the depth of silence, darkness, and retreat. They bring us to the deepest states of relaxation.

Herbs that heal and balance the water element often work on the reproductive system and the sacral chakra and are also associated with the portal of the West. Plants that have a yin energy, including jasmine, peony root, and shatavari, help nourish the feminine nature within us. Emmenagogues and other womb tonics, such as red raspberry leaf, angelica, and nettles, promote the shedding of the uterine wall and bring on menstruation. Others, such as mugwort and black cohosh, are connected to the waning energies and release menstrual blood. Damiana, calendula, and ashwaganda are sacral chakra allies with a strong solar element and are used as male reproductive tonics.

Floral cleansing waters and herbal baths alchemize the healing element of water with plant spirits that infuse our intentions and prayers into the waters within and around us.

Immune tonics are herbs and formulas that strengthen the immune system and help us prepare for the Winter months, when colds and flus run rampant. Honoring the Fall as a time to prepare for the Winter, we dig up the medicinal roots to make healing tinctures and syrups that will give us strength and health for the darker months ahead.

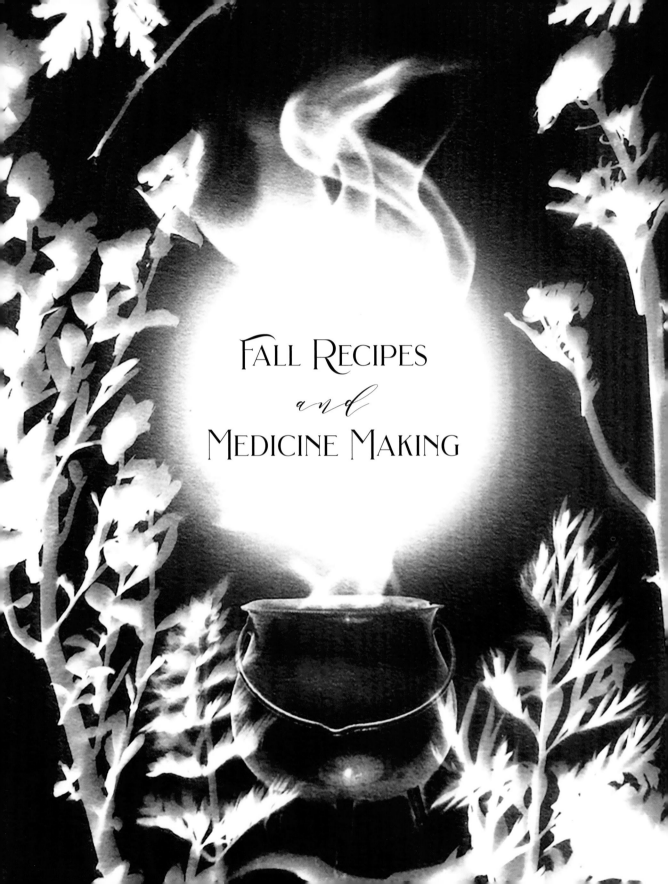

Fall Recipes

and

Medicine Making

Kava Bliss Elixir

Among my coven, I'm famous for this recipe, which draws upon the traditional alchemy of kava kava and coconut fat. It adds aphrodisiac herbs to enhance the blissful and sensual properties of the medicinal plants.

Enjoy the Kava Bliss Elixir to celebrate the end of your workday and your entrance into a relaxing and luxuriating evening. Enjoy it with a loved one, or alone to help awaken self-love and inspire rituals of pleasure and self-care. It's also a lovely way to end an intimate dinner party.

Yield: 1 serving

> 1 rounded teaspoon kava kava powder
> ½ teaspoon (1.2 g) ground cinnamon
> ¼ teaspoon (0.6 g) ground nutmeg
> Pinch ground cardamom
> 1 teaspoon (6.7 g) honey
> 1 tablespoon (15 g) coconut butter or 2 tablespoons (38 g) coconut cream
> Freshly grated nutmeg and/or dried rose petals for garnish (optional)

1. Blend all elixir ingredients with 8 oz (240 ml) of hot water in a high-speed blender until frothy.

2. Garnish with nutmeg and/or rose petals. Enjoy!

Kava Kava

Kava kava is a ceremonial drink. On the South Pacific islands of Vanuatu and Fiji, the roots were traditionally chewed and fermented in coconut. See pages 174 to 175 to learn more about this incredible plant and its many uses. This recipe is best for connecting to the pure presence of kava kava in the context of its alchemical and ancient relationship with coconut. This is how I prepare kava kava when I serve it for Kava Plant Meditations and to introduce people to this healing herb for the first time. This is also how I recommend people work with kava kava when retraining their nervous system.

Yield: 1 serving

> 2 tablespoons (14 g) kava kava powder (or more)
> 2 tablespoons (19 g) coconut cream

1. Stir the kava kava powder and 1 pint (473 ml) of spring water in a mason jar, cover, and leave overnight to infuse.

2. The following day, blend the kava kava mixture with the coconut cream in a high-speed blender until combined.

3. Serve at room temperature. Dose yourself according to your needs: you can sip it throughout the day to keep anxiety low and support mental focus or drink a big mug for a nice chill-out and full body and mind relaxation. Drink with others to open the heart and relax socially.

Kava-Cacao Seduction Elixir

As the name implies, this elixir brings us into a relaxed, euphoric state. It opens our heart, brings in pleasure and joy, and releases endorphins. The kava kava relaxes the body and releases tension, but the cacao has a more stimulating effect, making this elixir a wonderful potion to enjoy before making love, having a heart-to-heart conversation, or creating art into the evening hours.

Yield: 1 serving

> 8 oz (240 ml) hot water
> 1 rounded teaspoon (3 g) kava kava powder
> 1 tablespoon (5 g) cacao powder
> 1 teaspoon (7 g) maple syrup
> 1 tablespoon coconut butter (15 g) or
>   2 tablespoons (38 g) coconut cream
> Splash homemade vanilla extract (see right)
> ¼ teaspoon (1 g) maca powder (optional)
> Freshly grated nutmeg and/or dried rose
>   petals for garnish (optional)

1. Blend elixir ingredients in a high-speed blender until frothy.

2. Garnish with nutmeg and/or rose petals and enjoy!

Homemade Vanilla Extract

Making your own vanilla extract is easy and affordable, and you can ensure the ingredients are of the highest caliber. Like a tincture, the alcohol extracts the properties of vanilla over the course of 4 to 8 weeks.

Yield: 6 ounces (175 ml)

> 1 vanilla bean, split lengthwise and cut into
>   1-inch (2.5 cm) pieces
> 6 ounces (175 ml) bourbon, rum, vodka, or
>   other alcohol

1. Place the vanilla bean in an airtight jar and cover with alcohol. Close the jar tightly and shake.

2. Keep the jar in a dark cupboard for 4 to 8 weeks (or more) to infuse away from sunlight. Shake as often as you remember.

Fresh Willow Tea

Willow is a magickal tree that washes tension, tightness, pain and inflammation out of the body. When done correctly, harvesting her fresh shoots benefits her growth and makes the most delicious, heart-opening pink tea. A plant that opens us to the dreaming realms, she is a wonderful ally for meditation and a guide teaching us flexibility, how to bend and not break.

Yield: 1 serving

> Young willow shoots

1. Harvest young willow shoots. Skin the bark. Compost the outer bark. The most medicinal part is the inner green bark, the cambium layer.

2. Infuse a handful of green inner bark pieces in 1 quart (946 ml) hot water from the kettle for an overnight infusion, or bring bark to a simmer in a covered saucepan of 1 quart (946 ml) of water, so the medicine does not evaporate with the steam.

3. Drink warm or cold. Close your eyes and sip the tea for about 10 minutes, keeping your eyes closed and inviting in the spirit and medicine of the plant. Meditate on the sensations in your body and release any tension, grief, sorrow, pain, and prayers with the watery, healing release of willow washing through your emotional, physical, and spiritual body.

Willow Tincture

Willow tincture is wonderful medicine to have on hand in your apothecary as a pain reliever, antispasmodic, and gentle nervine. Willow tincture can offer relief for inflammation, arthritis, back pain, headaches, tension in the heart, stress, and more. Aspirin is derived from willow.

Yield: varies

> Fresh or dried inner green willow bark
> High-quality vodka or other alcoholic menstruum (or organic, non-GMO food-grade glycerin and spring water for nonalcoholic version)

1. If using the fresh inner green layer of willow bark, fill a jar of any size 90 percent full of bark pieces and top off with vodka. If using dried willow bark, fill a jar one-third full and top off with vodka. If making a nonalcoholic version, use a mixture of 80 percent glycerin and 20 percent spring water.

2. Seal with a lid, label, and store in a dark space for 8 weeks before straining and beginning to use.

3. Place 1 teaspoon (5 ml) of tincture in 4 ounces (120 ml) of water and drink to relieve cramps or pain, to open the heart, or for dreamtime.

Elder Immunity Cordial

This cordial is a go to when you want to keep sickness at bay. It is also delicious. You can dilute an ounce (28 ml) in a hot herbal tea or in warm water with a lemon wedge and a spoonful of honey and sip for strong dose of protection. As a mother, I am constantly surrounded by viruses and other illnesses that come home with my daughter from school. The moment I feel my immune system fighting something, I begin to take a tablespoon (15 ml) of this cordial every one to two hours. When sick, I also take a tablespoon that often, and it is incredible how quickly I am able to heal. The antiviral, antibacterial, and immune-boosting properties of this blend are incredibly powerful!

Yield: Approximately 1 quart (946 ml)

> 2 cups (256 g) dried elderflowers
> 2 cups (113 g) dried elderberries
> 3-inch (7.5 cm) chunk peeled and diced
>   fresh ginger root
> Fresh orange rind
> ½ cup (40 g) dried angelica root (optional)
> ½ cup (40 g) dried echinacea root
>   (optional)
> Sprig fresh thyme (optional)
> Brandy, to taste
> 1 cup (340 g) honey (optional)

1. Place dried ingredients in a quart-size mason jar. Top off with brandy.

2. Add honey, if using.

3. Serve 3 tablespoons (45 ml) in 3 ounces (90 ml) hot water and serve.

Nonalcoholic Elderberry Oxymel

Elderberry is a miraculous herb with powerful antiviral and immunostimulating properties. It is rich in Vitamin C and antioxidants, and it tastes delicious, which makes it a favorite for kids. This oxymel uses honey and vinegar as the menstruums of extraction, and thus it is alcohol free, safe for kids and folks who abstain from alcohol.

Yield: varies

> Dried elderberries
> Raw honey
> Apple cider vinegar

1. Fill a jar of any size 50 percent full of dried elderberries.

2. In a separate jar, prepare the menstruum by mixing equal parts raw honey and apple cider vinegar.

3. Pour the honey-vinegar solution into the jar of elderberries, filling it nearly to the top. Place a piece of waxed paper or plastic wrap over the mouth of the jar to prevent the vinegar and metal from touching. Seal the jar with the lid and shave.

4. Store away from light for 8 weeks, shaking as often as you remember.

5. Take 1 to 2 tablespoons (15 to 30 ml) every hour or two at the first sign of a cold. Take in similar doses when you are sick.

Dream Tea

This calming, relaxing, sweet, and demulcent tea feels like a dreamy, silky river. The marshmallow root, linden, and licorice make the tea slippery, hydrating, and mucilaginous, balancing the astringency of the willow. Dreamy and watery, you may drink this tea in the evening to unwind, release tension from the body, and relax the mind. Sip before bed and ask the plant spirits for dreams.

Yield: 1 serving

> 1 teaspoon (2 g) dried passion-vine leaf
> 1 teaspoon (0.6 g) linden leaf and flower
> ½ teaspoon (0.75 g) dried chamomile flowers
> ⅛ teaspoon (0.6 g) dried licorice root
> ½ teaspoon (0.75 g) dried willow bark
> ½ teaspoon (0.75 g) dried marshmallow root

1. Cover the dried ingredients with 8 ounces (240 ml) of hot water and let infuse for 20 minutes or more. Alternatively, bring to a simmer in a covered saucepan for a few minutes, so the medicine does not evaporate with the steam.

2. Strain and enjoy. You may sweeten it with honey, though the very small amount of licorice root brings sweetness without an overpowering taste of licorice.

Goodnight Goddess Mylk

The goddess who drinks this elixir will slip into the bliss of sleep nourished and embraced by the healing elixir. While ghee is made of butter, which can cause digestion issues, it is easily digestible. It's a medicinal food in Ayurvedic cuisine and herbalism.

Yield: 1 serving

> ¼ teaspoon (0.6 g) licorice root powder
> ½ teaspoon (1.1 g) ashwagandha powder
> ½ teaspoon (1.1 g) shatavari powder
> 1 tablespoon (12 g) ghee from grass-fed animals
> 1 teaspoon (6.7 g) raw honey
> Ground cinnamon, freshly grated nutmeg, and/or dried rose petals for garnish (optional)

1. Blend all mylk ingredients with 8 ounces (240 ml) of hot water in a high-speed blender until frothy.

2. Sprinkle cinnamon, nutmeg, or roses on top to garnish. Serve.

No-Bone Broth

This no-bone broth blend has become famous at my apothecary, Wild Love Apothecary, and within my community and home. You can decoct the ingredients for an hour or more to make a delicious broth. Serve it with a squirt of liquid aminos and a squeezed lemon wedge, poured over white rice or rice noodles with a handful of fresh cilantro. Add spice with red chile flakes and everyone will be licking their bowls, warming their bones, and deeply nourishing their immune reserves without overloading the digestive system. Or use it as a base for other soups, adding vegetables if you desire.

Yield: 1 gallon (3.8 L)

> 1 cup (48 g) dried chives
> ½ cup (56 g) burdock root
> ½ cup (56 g) dandelion root
> 2 slices reishi mushroom
> 1 cup (36 g) dried shiitake mushroom
> Salt, to taste

1. Place all the ingredients into 1 gallon (3.8 L) of water and bring to a boil.

2. Cover, lower the heat, and gently simmer on low for an hour or more until you get a strong decoction and broth.

3. Serve with liquid aminos, lemon, chile powder, as is or over rice noodles.

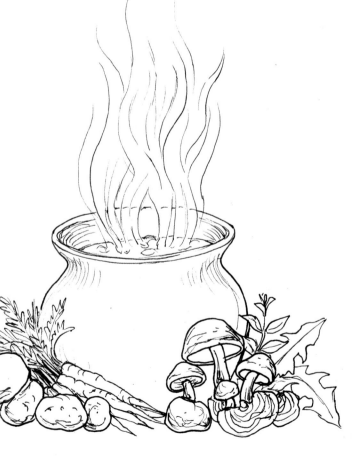

Simple Fall Veggie Soup Improv

Fall is the season of soups, which are deeply nourishing, grounding, and satiating yet cleansing and simple to digest. Here's a wonderful, versatile template for making your own with seasonal ingredients. I find that choosing one vegetable can make the soup delicious and not a mysterious bland medley. My favorites are broccoli, squash, and pumpkin. Everyone loves this creamy soup—it is so quick and easy to make, your guests will think it is magick!

Yield: varies

> Fall vegetable(s) of your choice
> 2 dried shiitake mushrooms
> 1 slice reishi mushroom
> Handful burdock root
> Water or vegetable broth (see sidebar
>   at right)
> A few tablespoons (30 g) butter or ghee
>   from grass-fed animals
> Salt to taste
> Ground black pepper to taste
> Turmeric, paprika, cumin, and/or other
>   spices to taste (optional)

1. Boil the vegetables in spring water or vegetable broth with the mushrooms and burdock root. The vegetables should be submerged by two inches of water or broth.

2. When the vegetables are soft, remove the reishi mushroom, which is too hard to blend.

3. Add the butter or ghee to taste and blend in a high-speed blender.

4. Season with salt and pepper. Add other seasonings to taste. Serve. You can store your broth for a few days in the fridge.

COMPOST VEGGIE BROTH

While the name is not appetizing, Compost Veggie Broth helps us remember that we can make a broth with the trimmings of our vegetables instead of composting them. When trimming off the tops or stems of celery, beets, carrots, broccoli, and other vegetables, save these nutritious chunks of in a container in the fridge. When you have a quart or more, cover in twice as much water as there are veggies, add salt, bring to a boil, cover, and simmer on low heat for an hour, making a mineral-rich broth. Use as a base for soups, sauces, curries, and other dishes within a couple of days.

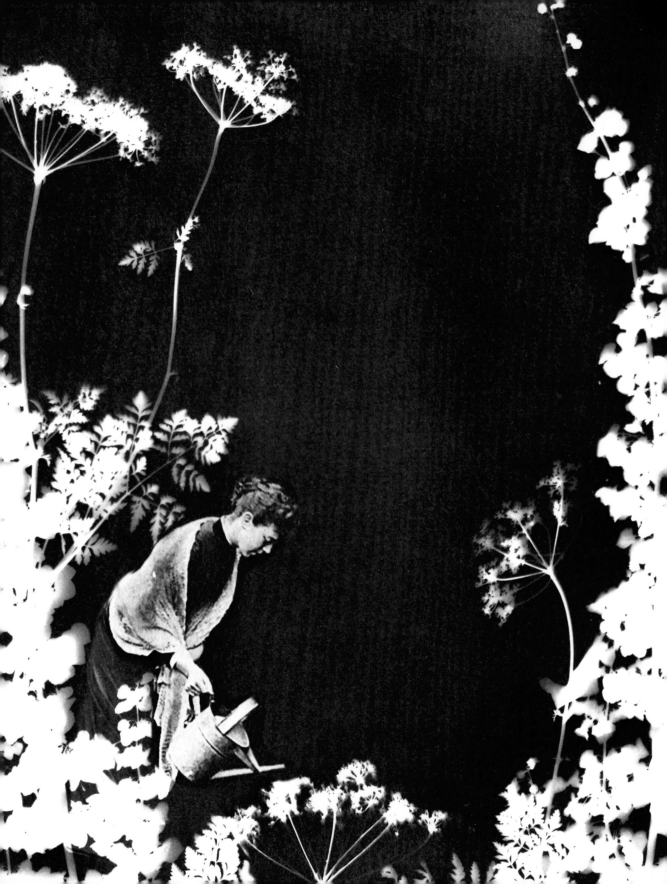

In the Garden, on the Earth

Fall is the start of the inbreath the Earth will be taking until the Spring Equinox. The waning energies bring the life-force energy of plants away from the aerial parts of their bodies and down into the roots and seeds that burrow into and fall to the ground.

In the Fall garden, the Green Witch digs up medicinal roots, including burdock, echinacea, ashwagandha, and marshmallow. Follow the sacred harvesting practices (see pages 34 to 35). Give ample space around the plant to dig and carefully work to get the whole root, not leaving large parts to break and rot in the Earth. Harvesting roots always feels vulnerable; unlike harvesting the aerial parts of a plant, this is the end of the life cycle for most medicinal root herbs. Fall is like that—it's a season that connects us to death, to vulnerability, to the tenderness of our heart, and to the thinning veil between life and death.

The Fall garden is a magickal portal for rituals of release and letting go. I cut back dead brush and twigs to create ritualistic bundles of tinder and fire starters so that which I release in the fall is consumed by the first fires of winter.

I weave prayers of letting go and release into my compost pile, deeply enjoying the smell of rotting leaves, the grounded feeling of the whole Earth slowing down and entering a period of reflection.

I spend time lying on the Earth, bringing my fiery spirit—so activated and burned out by the summer—into harmony with the waning Earth. I practice the Earth harmonizing ritual (page 91) as well as the Earth Whisper ritual (pages 170 to 171) often, winding myself down, dropping into the portals of fall in preparation for the deep dream of Winter.

I plan for the Earth to have a blanket of living green as she dreams, too. I pour large handfuls of sweet-pea seeds and fall cover crops on my naked belly and breasts, lie in the low Fall sun in my garden portal, and pray into the seeds that will sleep in her darkness and sprout new life.

I collect seeds from my garden and save, share, and trade them with friends. I caress seeds off of wild plants in the mountains and scatter them in the winds of change.

FALL RITUALS

Rituals of release, grief work, shamanic journeying, dream magick, herbal bathing,
flower waters, cord cutting, and midwifing death are some of the rituals of Fall.

Spiritually, the Fall invites us to dig deeper and engage what is at the root of our blossoming actions. Our transformation will not be complete without also composting the belief that productivity is more valuable than relaxation. The regenerative cycles of the wheel teach us to trust the eternal timing of nature. Through ritual we can cut away beliefs that push us into burnout and gently guide ourselves into a new way of being. We find that by entering the creative waters of the West, relaxing, resting, and cultivating nourishing connections, we awaken with greater inspiration, energy, genius, and stamina when it is time to do, create, expand, and produce!

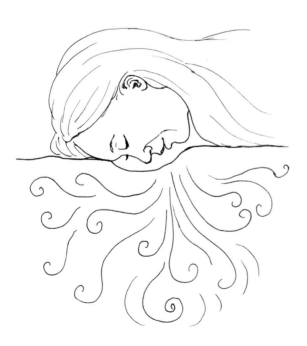

Earth Whisper Ritual

This is one of the my most beloved rituals, inspired by a ritual shared with me by a student. I haven't been able to trace the lineage of this ritual, however, and I have made some adaptations through the years. I share it with my apprentices each Fall, when we journey into our root chakras with the descending energies of Gaia. It is a profound ritual of release and renewal and an entry point for you to speak in great intimacy and connection into the fertile darkness of the Earth Mother's sacred flesh.

1. Always begin by harmonizing your body with the Earth (see page 91). Once you feel your body connected to the vibration of the Earth, lie with your belly on the Earth.

2. Smell the soil, close your eyes, and place your palms open on the ground around your face.

3. Speak to the Earth. Introduce yourself. Share your intention from your heart. Are you asking to release your burdens or speak your most sacred desires? Ask for permission to open the Earth's body.

4. Wait and listen for a yes. The Earth is the most generous and benevolent Mother. She is always available to take our burdens and griefs and transform them through her Self, but we must wait for permission.

5. When you feel a yes, dig a hole. I dig a hole that is big enough for my mouth and nose to fit into with my brow or third eye resting on the Earth.

6. Speak out loud to the Mother from your vulnerable places into her open body. This is an incredible and sacred practice. To release burdens, speak your grief, releasing what weighs heavy on your heart. Ask the Mother to take it from you. Thank her.

When releasing energy, we offer intention into the space that has been made. You do not need to go into detail or call specific things in, although you can also pray in that way if you wish. But do consider that there is an energetic void. Fill it with trust, love, and your prayers.

7. Give a gift to the Mother—perhaps a strand of hair, water, a flower mandala, or sacred herbs. If it's something meaningful that's a little difficult to give away, then it is a true gift.

8. Ask forgiveness for opening her up in this way. Thank her for her generosity.

9. Close the hole. Lie, breathe, journal, and integrate.

Cord-Cutting Ritual

This ritual was taught to me by Sweet Medicine Nation, a medicine teacher and elder. I have adapted it and continue to work with it when I feel energetic cords entangling my spirit, emotional body, or heart and it is time to let go. We often say we are done with bad habits, tendencies, or relationships, but an embodied ritual delivers the message to our whole soul, all of our cells, and the Great Web of what is seen and unseen. This is a powerful ritual for releasing old cords.

1. Go into a forest with a heart full of prayer, prepared and clear, ready to release. Bring a knife, a long string (such as the ones used for friendship bracelets), and offerings. Create sacred space.

2. Cast from your heart the prayer and request for a tree to call you forth—the tree that is willing to assist you in this release. When you feel the connection, go barefoot to the tree and harmonize your energy with it. You may do so by using the Earth harmonizing ritual (page 91), laying your body against the trunk, or meditating with it.

3. Spend some time, breathe deeply, ground your energy, and open your heart. Speak to the tree as you would to an elder—with respect, from a humble heart, sharing that you wish to release old cords. Explain why and how ready you are to release.

4. Ask permission to work with the tree in this ritual, make an offering to the tree, and listen for the answer.

5. If you feel a yes, stand before the tree, bare feet on the Earth. Tie the string around your waist, speaking out loud what it represents. Tie the other end around the trunk of the tree.

6. Lean back gently, with your hand on the taut string, and feel the cords. Speak what the cords are, imagining the energies that bind you entering into the string. Lift your blade and affirm out loud, "I cut these cords and am free of them now and forevermore."

7. Cut the string. Close your eyes and feel the energetic shift in your body. Ground your energy by sitting, placing your palms or lying belly down on the Earth, or leaning against the tree. Take a moment. Allow for the release. Feel the difference in your body.

8. Give gratitude, thank the tree, and open the sacred circle you had cast, thanking the spirits. Leave the string around your waist until it naturally falls off. Notice when it falls away.

Grieving with Water and Red Clover

Grieving is an important part of opening to life, love, and renewal. When we do not properly grieve something, a "stuckness" and density can stay in us and we can become depressed or ill. We do not grieve in order to feel better (although properly grieving almost always makes us then feel lighter and more open); we grieve in order to move energy and transform. Likewise, we do not grieve in order to not be brokenhearted, but grieving does allow energy to move and the heart to continue its own destiny of transformation and mysterious unfoldment.

Grieving is a watery thing. In the Fall, when the portals of water are open, I often feel nostalgia and access the currents of grief for no particular reason. Fall is indeed an optimal time to release energy with tears and through rituals of grief.

To open the portals of moving grief, give yourself uninterrupted time and, ideally, access to nature. Ready a journal, warm tea, a blanket, and the option to rest after a release and replenishing. If you feel that you have something or someone to grieve but your tears or the energy is stuck, I recommend working with moving water. A river is a wonderful ally, but a shower will do as well. You can call upon the heart-opening, water-moving spirit of red clover for assistance.

Prepare an infusion of red clover blossoms by placing a large handful of the dried blossoms in quart-sized jar and topping it off with hot water. Infuse for an hour or more. Create sacred space, burn blessing herbs, and light candles in your bathroom. Play music that softens your heart and shifts your consciousness. Meditate, drinking the red clover, speaking to her spirit and asking her for help in releasing. Speak to her like you would to a grandmother and allow for moments of

listening to her energy in your body, receiving. Breathe and soften. Anoint your brow, gently wash your skin with her infusion, and pray. Notice when you feel called to get into a shower or warm bath, and ask the water to cleanse you of the energy that has been stuck and is ready to release. If you take a bath, drain it without leaving it when you're finished, feeling the water and energy draining away, going back into the Earth. Open up the sacred container and thank the spirits.

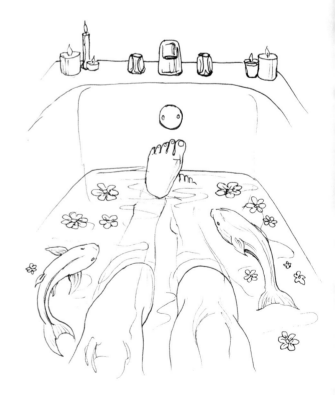

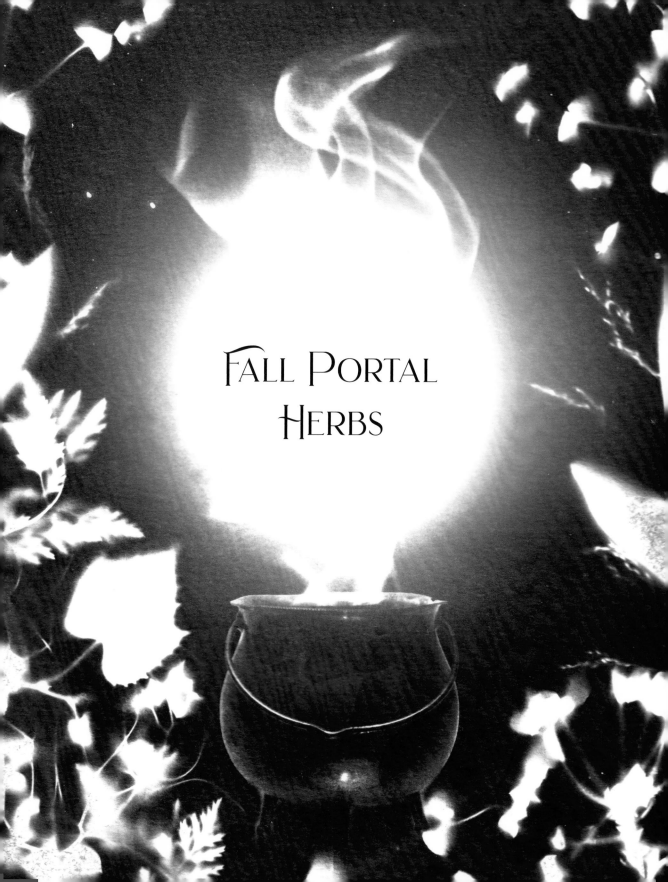

Fall Portal Herbs

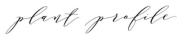

plant profile
Kava Kava

LATIN NAME *Piper methysticum*

FAMILY Piperaceae

Kava kava (or simply kava) is a shrub with heart-shaped leaves growing in humid, tropical lands of the Pacific Islands of Hawaii and Fiji; it's native to Vanuatu. An ancient herb of profound cultural and ceremonial significance, it's called the root of happiness and has been used for centuries. It's currently only propagated by hand.

HERBAL AND MEDICINAL PROPERTIES

- Deeply relaxing and mildly euphoric: a consciousness-shifting, profound teacher plant that has shared much wisdom about how to bring the modern human back into balance
- Sedative, nervine: ally for anxiety, public speaking, and social engagements as well as to help unwind after a busy day, relaxing the nerves and the body; deeply calming and relaxing, it aids in sleep and with insomnia without drowsiness, letting you wake up feeling renewed
- Antispasmodic and anti-inflammatory: ally to help the spirit ground into the body after a physical trauma; upon drinking, there is a gentle numbing sensation in the mouth and mucous membranes and a warm tingle through the body that is deeply relaxing and helpful for cramps and pain
- Antidepressant: uplifting to the spirit, opening to the heart and mind
- Bitter and carminative: moves energy in the digestive system and solar plexus
- Ally for self-love and self-acceptance

PLANT SPIRIT HEALING

The spirit of kava in meditation often begins by grounding the body, allowing our roots to relax into the supportive Earth below, connecting us to gravity, releasing tension from the body, and washing away cramps, tightness, pain, and inflammation. What a wonderful feeling to drop into such blissful relaxation and presence! The mind follows, becoming calmer, and the spirit of the plant often says, "Relax. Everything is just fine." Our human worries begin to seem small, and an ancient connection to deep time and the greater scheme of things enters the energetic body. The body feels safe, and the human spirit is able to enter the body more deeply—this is profoundly healing for those who experienced some kind of physical trauma to their body, such as a car accident or other injury or violence. Kava can heal the relationships between the mind, spirit, and body, retraining our nervous system so our spirit learns that it is safe and good to be here, embodied. This does long-term wonders for those who are prone to anxiety, tend to leave their body, and are humming at the vibration of fear or nervousness. The hum of kava is deep, yummy, slow, and lubricating. It sings its base notes into our bones, waters, flames, and the space between our cells. Once we have dropped into a deep state of relaxation, the spirit often connects us to our creative center, sacral chakra, center of pleasure while opening the third eye. Kava has given me profound guidance throughout my life about a large matter of subjects, one of which is how to birth things into the world. The spirit of kava taught me that everything we create has a spirit, and the vibration in which that thing in question was created continues to vibrate out in rippling remnants of the frequency in which it was created. Therefore, if we create something from a place of chaos, urgency, fear, or the like, our creation, no matter how great its intended purpose, will continue rippling an aspect of that vibration out into the world. And so, what we birth can create more chaos and noise, or, if we begin by harmonizing our energetic body and then birth from deep trust, rooted calm, and embodied bliss, can create more harmony. Our creations can be medicine simply by being and existing. As I guide people into connection with the spirit of kava, I see how this plant is a profound healer for the overstressed, overwhelmed, overstimulated modern human. Kava weaves us into community, a nonhierarchical circle; it drops us into our heart and harmonizes us to deep trust.

PRECAUTIONS

Overall kava is generally considered safe, even for use with children. It's not recommended during pregnancy, however, as its antispasmodic properties can relax the uterus. Also, kava is possibly taxing on the liver with long-term use.

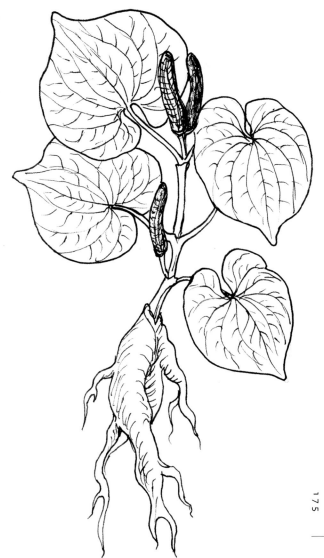

plant profile
Willow

LATIN NAME *Salix* spp.

FAMILY Salicaceae

The magickal willow shrubs and trees have alternating, usually narrow leaves and catkins, often with a silver underside that glistens in the moonlight, near the streams and wild waters and lands where she loves to grow. Many species of willow can be found throughout the Northern Hemisphere in Europe, Asia, and North America. She often holds banks of rivers, supporting other plants with the rooting hormones that she releases into shared water systems. She dies back each Fall to be reborn in the Spring, an ally of regeneration. With thousands of years of recorded history of magick, lore, and medicine, she is found in stories and apothecaries of many diverse cultures and lands and is often woven into myths of the moon, the Goddess, and the Witch.

HERBAL AND MEDICINAL PROPERTIES

- Analgesic (pain relieving) and anti-inflammatory: a wonderful ally for arthritis, headaches, cramps, and any pains or injuries to the musculoskeletal system, including inflammation in joints
- Teaches us to be like her branches physically and spiritually: flexible, able to bend and not break
- Febrifuge, antiseptic: a remedy for colds and fevers
- Bitter: supports metabolism and digestion
- Astringent: useful topically and internally for clearing and tonifying skin

HERBAL AND MEDICINAL PROPERTIES

Willow is a powerful, deep, feminine, and mystical plant spirit that can wash away tightness, stuck energy, hurt, and grief from the emotional body. Calling her in, we begin to feel our body relax and soften, cradled in a basket of her willow embrace. There, a gentle stream washes our hearts and souls clean, singing songs to the deep parts of our inner mysteries and dreams. She can teach us how to love more deeply, how to enter profound presence and other realms. She is a healer and a guide, and meditating with her gives our hearts the opportunity to ask for guidance in relationships and life. She reminds us that each death leads to new life, and though she goes dormant in the Fall, her presence is felt in deep time, in the void. She can take us there, helping us ride currents of regeneration, teaching us to flow with grace, flexibility, and wisdom on the river of life. She weaves community and supports other plants in her ecosystem, reminding us we are never alone.

FAVORITE USES

- Fresh or dried willow tea
- Meditating with willow in nature, asking for guidance, prayer work
- As tincture for pain and inflammation
- Weaving baskets of willow

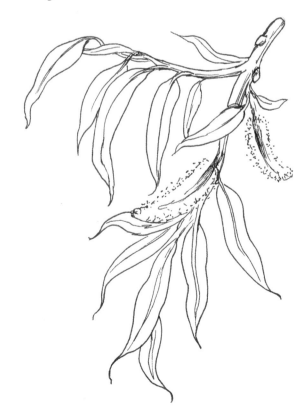

plant profile

Elder

LATIN NAMES *Sambucus nigra, Sambucus canadensis*

FAMILY Adoxaceae

A deciduous tree or shrub with many trunks, varieties of elder grow worldwide in forests, meadows, and even urban areas with disturbed soil. In the summer, elder is crowned with clusters of thousands of sweet-scented, cream-colored blossoms, which then turn to clumps of small, dark-purple elderberries, beloved by birds and healers alike. Deeply woven into folk medicine, magick, and the lore of diverse lands and cultures, elder holds the gateway to the fairy realm in Celtic and European pagan traditions. The leaves are toxic, the flowers and berries are medicinal, and the wood is magickal for wands, ritual brooms, or clapping stick instruments made by the Chumash Native Americans.

HERBAL AND MEDICINAL PROPERTIES

- Children's ally for fevers and sickness; diaphoretic
- Stimulates the immune system; wonderful remedy and incredibly effective in protecting from and healing the flu, colds, viruses, and respiratory infections
- Relaxing to tissue, lightly antispasmodic, and soothing to digestion

PLANT SPIRIT HEALING

I can easily drink a quart of elderflower infusion to ward off a cold, but when I meditate with elderflower tea, only a few sips in, I feel the plant spirit entering so strongly that sometimes I become nauseous with the amount of cosmic and heavenly energy this plant spirit grounds into the body and earth. The spirit of lighting is felt with the plant; frequencies from upper realms travel through it to our Earth plane. I can understand why elder has been used in magick and shamanically to bridge and access the realm of the fay. I find the plant spirit to be very protective and useful in banishing negative energies and protecting the auric field of healers, children, and anyone who wishes to seek

assistance from higher realms. I often gift elderflowers to mamas with babies for a bath—elder loves children, and the spirit of the plant feeds their guardian angels.

FAVORITE USES

- Elderflower or elderberry tea
- Immunity cordial and syrups (see recipes, page 164)
- Elderflower champagne
- Elderflower herbal washes and ritual baths
- Plant-spirit meditation in wild nature
- Magickal broomsticks and wands made of straight suckers and new shoots

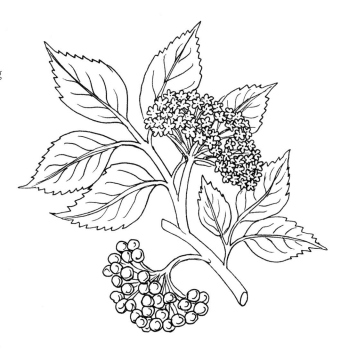

plant profile

Passionflower

LATIN NAME *Passiflora incarnata*

FAMILY Passifloraceae (passionflower family)

Passionflower is a beautiful vine with twirling tendrils, cosmic, starlike flowers, deeply lobed green leaves, and edible fruit. Native to the southern United States (Virginia, Texas, and Tennessee) and to Central and South America, it is now extensively cultivated in Europe, notably in Italy, as well as elsewhere in North America. The leaves, vines, and flowers are used for medicine, and the fruit is delicious and rich in vitamins and antioxidants.

HERBAL AND MEDICINAL PROPERTIES

- Indigenous people of the Americas, including the Aztecs, first used passion vine for fruit and as a sedative to treat insomnia and anxiety; colonizers then took the plant back to Spain, where it became an integral part of European herbal medicine.
- Nervine and gentle sedative: a prized remedy for insomnia, anxiety, nervousness, and tension in the body
- Mild aphrodisiac and antidepressant: opening to the heart chakra and sacral chakra
- Consciousness shifter: a wonderful ally for meditation, art, creativity, and dreaming

PLANT SPIRIT HEALING

Passion vine relaxes the mind and body, opens the heart, and lifts us up to the heavens, just as the vines reach to the sky with cosmic flowers that look like spiraling crown chakras. The spirit of this plant connects us to self-love, confidence, and beauty. Healing to the solar plexus, she calms anxiety, negative self-talk, and fear of sensuality. She often comes to me as a magickal, shape-shifting feminine spirit that opens the third eye and can take us on a shamanic journey—especially helpful in reclaiming one's creative energy and for matters of the heart.

FAVORITE USES

- Fresh or dried passion vine tea for evening relaxation, art making, dream time
- Meditating with the tea, asking for guidance, prayer work, shamanic journeying
- Flower essence
- As tincture for anxiety and sleep
- Contemplating her incredible, otherworldly flowers
- In designing gardens, I plant her over arbors to create shade, beauty, and provide ample medicine and food.
- Her fruits are delicious in drinks and desserts.

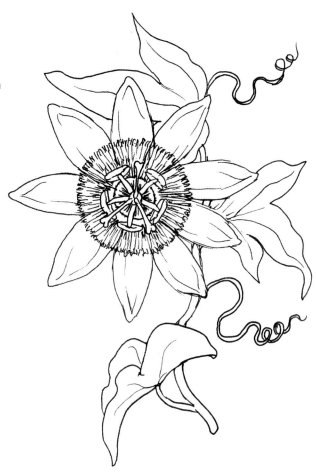

plant profile

Linden, Lime Flower

LATIN NAME *Tilia × europaea*

FAMILY Tiliaceae/Malvaceae (linden family)

Linden is a deciduous grandmother tree growing to 100 feet (30.5 meters). It has smooth gray bark, heart-shaped leaves, and clusters of pale yellow flowers that smell like honey and jasmine, swarm with bees, and drip nectar in the summer. Linden grows in the temperate Northern Hemisphere in Europe, North America, and Asia in wild areas as well as in cities. It has been used in herbal folk medicine since ancient times.

HERBAL AND MEDICINAL PROPERTIES

- Nervine, antispasmodic, anti-inflammatory: calms anxiety, stress, and tension in the mind, body, musculoskeletal system, and tissue of the heart, opening the heart chakra, nourishing and grounding the root, and bringing balance to the air element in the body

- Diaphoretic: used for fevers and colds, safe for children and elderly alike

- Mild expectorant: opens breath and lungs

- Calming and nourishing to the heart: lowers blood pressure and relieves anxiety in the heart, belly, mind, or anywhere else it gets stored

- Gently cleansing, supporting digestion and soothing the belly

PLANT SPIRIT HEALING

Linden is my beloved grandmother. When drinking her and calling her in, we immediately feel our soul, heart, and body relax, falling into the arms of the most divine, benevolent, sweet, grounded grandmother. There we can cry, release, rest, and pray. Linden is a magickal tree with ancient threads of legends and lore, and it is considered sacred and protective against evil spirits. In Christianity, the tree is dedicated to the Blessed Virgin; in Poland, many shrines to the Mother Mary are hung on her trunk.

When everything feels lost and you find yourself in times of despair, heartbreak, or grief, call on sweet linden to hold and heal you. Drink and meditate with her tea anytime you wish to connect to the energies of the divine Mother and the highest vibrations of feminine love. She is healing to those who need mothering and to caretakers who give so much and could use some receiving and rest. An ally to pray to those who have passed, opening the heart, third eye, and crown. Linden has taught me about vibrational medicine and healing frequencies. She once explained to me that we are all like wooden string instruments and that life will move through our bodies, playing us, creating sound vibration. It is our responsibility to tune our instrument each day so that as life greets us in all of her unexpected ways, we create harmonic frequencies and healing songs. She showed me that beginning each day in meditation with her tea is one way of tuning our instrument and heart to the vibration of unconditional love.

FAVORITE USES

- Hot overnight infusion, drunk cold the following day (drink often)

- To wind down, relax, and soften the heart

- To assist in open-hearted communication with a lover or friend

- To work with ancestors, guides, and angels

- Grief work, healing heartbreak, rituals of release and meditation

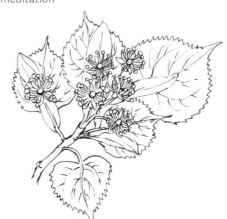

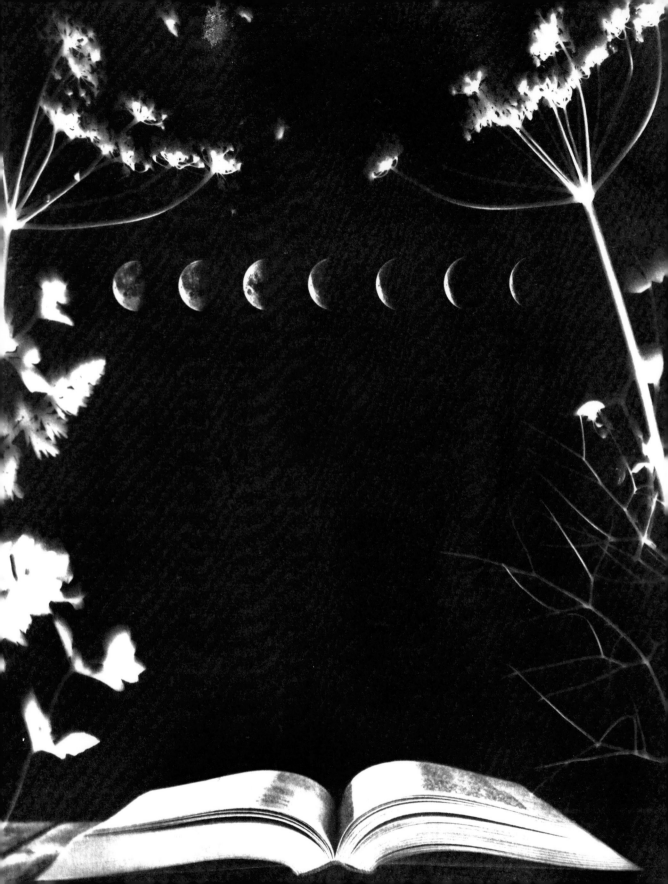

West Portal Journal Prompts

Reflect on the element of water in you.

Water element in balance:

- Feeling to heal—not escaping from pain and emotions but entering them as portals with calm wisdom and grounded trust in your ability to hold and nourish yourself (healthy earth). Knowing the medicine is in the wound.

- Deep intuition, psychic abilities, embodied guidance and knowing

- Shamanic practice, journeying, divination tools, wisdom, and depth

- Empathy and compassion; unconditional love that heals (all elements in balance)

- Creativity, grace, artistic movement, dance

- Flexibility and ability to go with the flow while staying centered in the Self

- Healthy boundaries, self-love, self-care (balanced with earth and fire)

Water element out of balance:

- Being overly emotional (usually needs more earth or fire)

- Being wishy washy, unclear, inconsistent; lacking of direction (usually needs earth or fire)

- Flax tissue, losing liquid and chi, such as postpartum (needs more earth or water)

- Dry tissue, being brittle physically or emotionally (needs more water)

- Hyperactivity, restlessness, being controlling (needs more water)

Reflect on how you can nourish your inner Wise Woman archetype in your journal:

- What can you give more death to, in order to create more life in moons to come?

- What is dead and asking to be released?

- How can you make your load lighter?

- How can you alchemize the fruits of your labor and slow down enough to savor the offerings of your creations? How can they feed you for months to come at the time of nondoing?

- How can you prepare for the Winter?

- What roles and responsibilities can you release?

- What awakens your sensuality, creativity, and imagination?

- What are your hands asking for? Would they like to make something?

- What self-care practices bring you into deeper bliss and help you enter a restorative state?

- Which creative projects feel nourishing and can be your priority as you slow down your expectations of doing?

- How can you do less and be more?

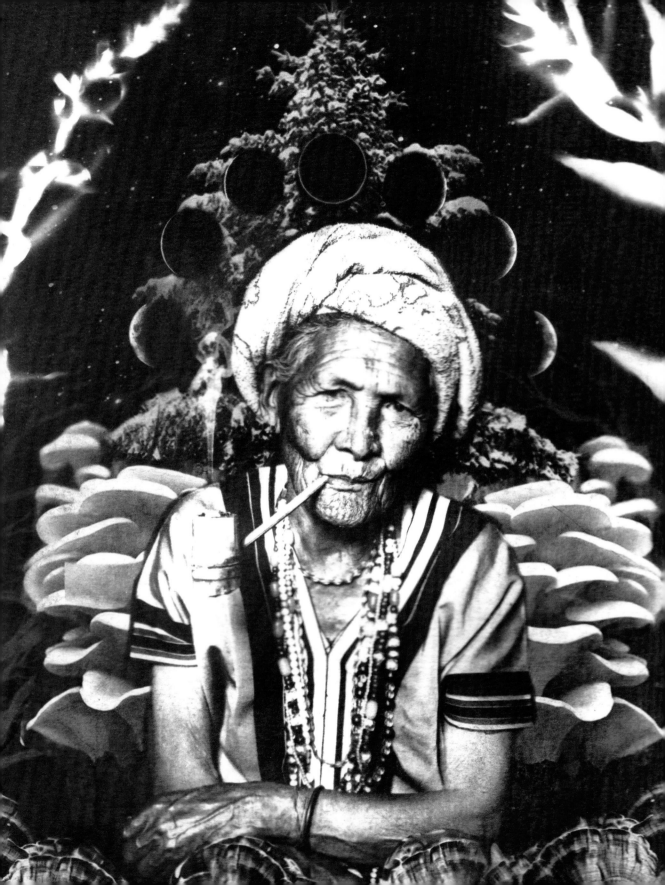

Chapter 7

EARTH MAGICK & MEDICINE OF WINTER

Release & Rest: Dream & the Void | North · Earth · The Crone

The Portal of the North at a Glance

ELEMENT Earth

TIME OF DAY Night | 10:00 p.m.–4:00 a.m.

MOON PHASE Dark

SEASON OF SOLAR YEAR Winter | December, January, February

EARTH HOLY DAYS Yule (Winter Solstice) | February 2

WHEEL OF LIFE ARCHETYPE Crone | Age: 64+

ENERGIES Dormant, still, void consciousness, the hag, the hermit, solitude, otherworldly, nondoing, recovery, rest

HEALING HERBS

Nervines and sedative herbs Hops, kava kava, blue vervain

Adaptogenic, wisdom, and longevity herbs Reishi, eleuthero, chaga, gotu kola, ashwagandha, tulsi

Dreaming herbs, third eye openers Mugwort, blue lotus, passion vine

Medicinal Mushrooms Reishi, chaga, lion's mane, turkey tail, shiitake, maitake

TENDING THE GARDEN The garden sleeps under mulch or rests under cover crops

APOTHECARY Taking shamanic journeys to inquire what kind of medicine wants to be made right now; Winter is often the time to make medicine for immunity and warding off infection with dried herbs, or double extractions of medicinal mushrooms.

RITUALS Rituals of rest, sleep, shamanic journeying; drumming, Aat making, journaling, reading; rituals of tending fire and flame; if need be, drawing on rituals from the South portal to keep the fires burning— lovemaking, cacao medicine, friction fire

Gaia Speaks

Shhhhhhhhh.

It is Winter. It is dark.

Stay still.
Silent.
Listen.

Snow muffles sound
and we dream,
hibernating in the folds of the Earth mother's flesh.

Find your cave.
Enter the portal.

Dark moon
like a womb,
the fertile void.

All things come from here and
to her darkness will return.
To die and be reborn
again and again.

In this moment, we pause
between inbreath and exhale,
between death and rebirth.

The void
no thing
deep dream
of renewal

Dissolve.

Dissolve into me.
Let your bones exhale into the decomposing soil below.
Let your mind spill like black ink into the night sky.

Become one with the Great Mystery.

In the moments of merging,
the Great Dream will enter the threads of your web.

And when you awaken,
you will be pregnant with the Great Song humming
in your cells and the spaces in between.

In all of your secret places.
The primordial sound,
you an instrument,
tuned
to the song of creation.

Humm my humm
Of deep time.
Timeless.
No time.
Rest.

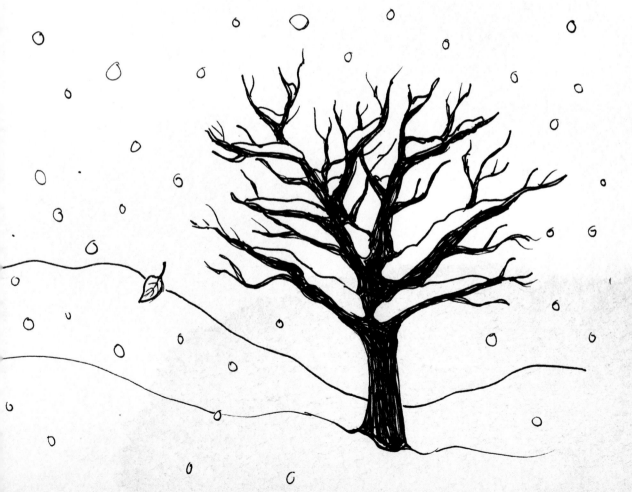

Rest to Regenerate Yourself, Dark Crone

It is Winter. It is dark. This is not the time of doing. This is the time of dreaming and dissolving our consciousness into the fertile void from which all life comes and into which all life returns. There is renewal here, through stopping what you are doing and dropping deep into being in oneness with all that is. It is the pause in between breaths. It is suspension. It is the deep sleep when we dissolve into the dream of Gaia and remember not what occurred upon waking. From this time, we arise renewed. But the renewal itself is part of the mystery. And to enter the void, we must be willing to dissolve ourselves completely, offering ourselves to realms unknown. To merge our consciousness with the dark moon and the starry sky. To drop our body into the rest of hibernating animals that sleep in the caves and folds of the Earth Mother's flesh. Humbling ourselves as we bow before the vastness of all we do not know, we become wiser and more whole.

Now is the time of the Crone. The old hag—wrinkled by time and experience, with a twinkle of magic in her eyes—has one foot beyond the veil. She is wild and fierce and deep in her love and sovereignty. She cares not about fitting in. She expands beyond the human realms and limitations of this Earthly plane. Her pull is the spiral of the galaxies, the dreams in the darkness, the singing over bones. She looks not for a lover or companion; done are her days of raising children and building matter. She belongs to the time of dissolving, her mind in the song of her rattle. She is mystic. She is hermit. In a healthy and whole society, there are those who honor and care for her, bring her food, seek her counsel, humble themselves to her wisdom, sweep her stoop, and warm her bones, so she can come and go, with or without (in or outside of) body. A whole culture holds space where she is allowed to be "crazy," to be misunderstood. The flickers of clarity we may gather from her words are like a strand of pearls, of equal value to the velvet darkness in between each bead, which we will never grasp or understand. There is space for not knowing—here we learn to bow before the Great Mystery.

We enter our Crone time in the dark time of the night, in the deepest of sleep. We enter the portal with the dark moon each month and at the longest nights of the year in Winter. When we bleed our menses and connect to the dark moon, we are in our crone aspect—at our most psychic, with one foot in between realms. If we can release the worldly realms at this time and have our bones warmed and stoops

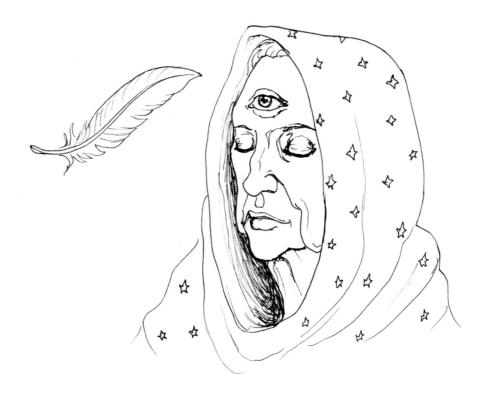

swept, we can travel into mystical realms and cultivate our inner Crone even when linear age has us young and bleeding. These portals open to us. There is value in developing a relationship with all aspects of the whole, including our inner hag. While the gateway of the darkness and void consciousness is most secret and often feared or rejected, it is from this very fertile nothingness that the first spark of life emerges. Without death, there is no life.

"Die before you die," said the Prophet Muhammad. In the portal of the North, we learn how to die. Here we dissolve. Here we become wise by realizing we know nothing at all. And we practice and get better at surrender, at bowing before the Great Mystery, at releasing control, at dying. Over and over and over again.

Rest to regenerate yourself,
dark Crone.

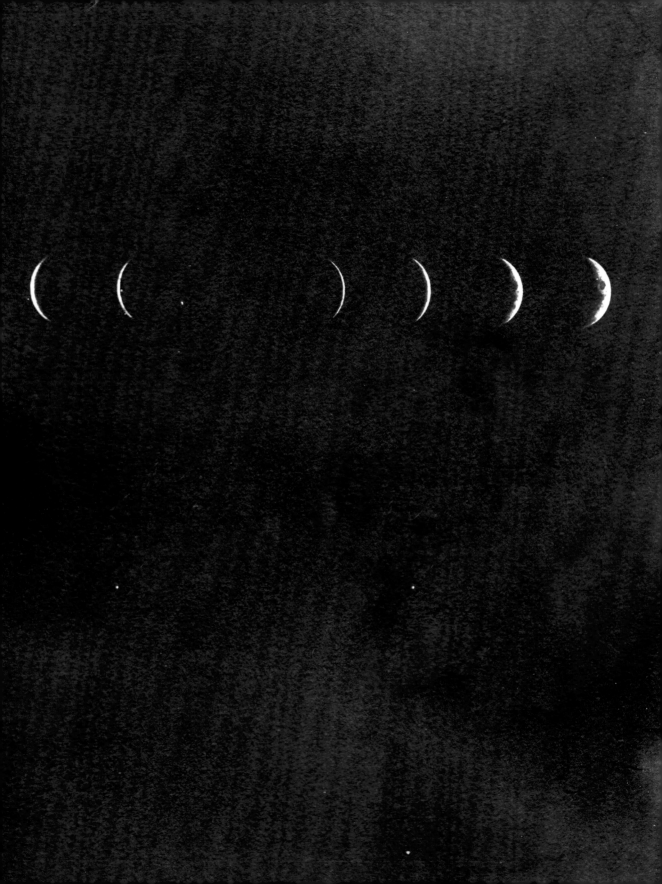

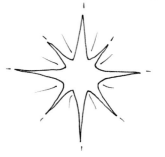

Entering the Portals of the North

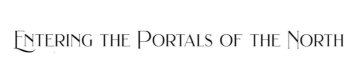

The portal of the North is the void of darkness through which Nature's energy passes to be fully released in the fertile darkness and emerge renewed. It is a mysterious moment of "in between": the pause between breaths, the disappearing of the moon, the longest night of the year, the deaths we die before we die, and then the final death of our body, which releases our energy and soul in a way that none of us fully understand.

In the solar year, the season of Winter connects us to the energy of the Northern portal, spanning the months of December, January, and February in the Northern Hemisphere, with the Winter Solstice (December 20–23) marking the official start of Winter. It's the longest night of the year, the portal of darkness, when many cultures pray for the rebirth of the sun. In the wheel of our lives, the North corresponds to the archetype of the Crone—the hag, hermit, and mystic.

We arrive in the Winter after releasing worldly obligations and linear doings in the Fall, becoming lighter and more fluid so we can dissolve into the void consciousness and merge with the Great Mystery. Our only work is to unravel ourselves so that we can drop deeply into restorative rest and deep sleep. There we enter the slow brain waves, which renew cells and bring harmony to our body functions.

Spiritually, in this state of deep rest, we dissolve our ego consciousness and our separate sense of self into the fertile darkness. In the moment of oneness with the fertile void, something mysterious and utterly magickal occurs: we become pregnant with the dream of Gaia. After this merging with the void consciousness, we begin to stir awake and bring our energy back to ourselves, awakening our boundaries of Self. Only this time, a part of the Great Mystery remains in us—an energetic imprint of the dream that Gaia is dreaming into being. This dream becomes a seed. As the energies of the year begin to wax, we journey into the moment of the first spark of Imbolc, where we often begin to feel sensations that echo the journey of becoming aware we are pregnant with child. When a woman physically becomes aware she is pregnant, she revels in the sensations and does not begin to assume who the child will be—it is too early to tell. In this case, we are spiritually pregnant with a seed that will grow through the unique flame and fire of our Self and blossom into Spring creations and Summer gifts, through us, for the world. It is too early to vision what we will birth. It is time to be in awe of the stirring inside, knowing it comes from beyond the construct of a human mind. Dissolving ourselves into the Winter portal allows us to birth creations and ride regenerative waves much greater than anything our small humanness could ever devise. In places that are largely unconscious and richly mysterious, we draw on waves of energy that crescendo through us as we wax with luminous moon, rise with the sap of the Spring trees, and bud with the apple blossoms.

Entering the North Each Night

In the twenty-four-hour wheel of the day, North corresponds to the nighttime and optimal hours of sleep, roughly from 10:00 p.m. to 4:00 a.m. The yin energies of relaxation of the Western portal carry us into deeply restorative rest at night.

If we have moved through the portal of the West in harmony, we will effortlessly slip into the North. The nervines we work with in the evening to help our minds and nerves unwind from the business of the day help us relax and get deeper sleep. Stronger doses of nervines or working with sedatives helps with insomnia or light sleeping. On the other hand, if we do not use the evening hours of the West to unwind and relax, and rather continue working right until we go to sleep, we are more likely to "crash" and then wake up in the middle of the night. The medicine of the North portal is regenerative sleep, during which our bodies heal, create human growth hormone, regenerate, and come into balance. Deep rest is imperative for our longevity.

Night Tools to Help You Enter Deep Realms of Restorative Rest

- Take a bedtime nervine or sedative tea or Kava Bliss Elixir (see page 161) before going to bed.

- Take a hot bath before going to bed.

- Have a massage.

- Meditate, pray, or do shamanic journeying.

- Avoid pollution in your bedroom, using blackout curtains if need be.

- Turn off electronics in your bedroom.

- Avoid screen time for at least thirty minutes (but ideally two hours) before bedtime.

- Use an app that reduces the blue light of your screens.

- Use aromatherapy for sleep, such as a lavender pillow, chamomile, or smudging your room (see pages 30 to 31).

- Place a salt lamp by your bedside.

- Perform your nightly rituals by candlelight.

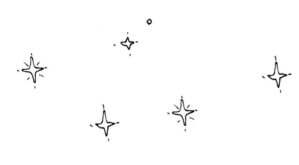

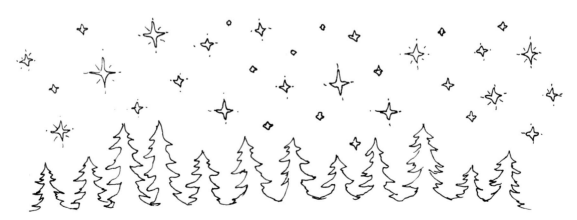

Resting with the Dark Moon

This magnificent refuge is inside you.
Enter.
Shatter the darkness that shrouds the doorway.
Be bold. Be humble.
Put away the incense and forget
The incantations they taught you.
Ask no permission from the authorities.
Close your eyes and follow your breath
To the still place that leads to the
Invisible path that leads you home.

—St. Theresa of Avila

The moment of the dark moon corresponds to true North and the longest night of the year at the Winter Solstice. In the lunar cycle, the few days on either side of the dark moon take us into the energies of this portal. However, it is truly the one night of the dark moon that is most potent for the spiritual and energetic merging with the fertile darkness.

For menstruating women, the first day of the moon cycle corresponds to the dark moon. The days of bleeding are their Winter and time of rest. According to a tradition of Chinese medicine many thousands of years old, a woman should truly rest, preferably in bed, drinking warm teas and broths, while she is menstruating for four days. It is hard for the modern woman to successfully take up this practice, but it is also one of the most ancient and effective strategies for healing hormonal imbalances, reducing the duration of length of bleeding, and reducing cramps and PMS in future cycles. It is also a phenomenal tool for aligning

us with our body's ability to regenerate itself. Women who begin this practice complete their cycle feeling revived and renewed, bursting with a new Spring-like energy. Some who maintain it have reported significant physical and energetic regeneration—feeling and looking more youthful!

Although it is easy to dismiss this practice as unrealistic, I suggest you throw that limiting belief into the cauldron of transformation and actually try it. A dear friend of mine did, while her identical twin dismissed it as impossible due to the demands of modern life. My friend used the Fall portal of her cycle to prepare for her Winter bleeding time—making soups and broths, arranging playdates and sitters so she could have alone time, and canceling appointments so she could stay home in bed. After a few months, not only did she find she had a tremendous amount of energy each Spring of her cycle, but people began to think she was younger than her twin. The physical, emotional, and spiritually regenerative effects of this ancient practice were impossible to deny. Now they both make it a priority to rest for four days during their moon time.

The bleeding woman will connect to the Winter portal during her menstrual cycle as well as during the dark moon of the lunar cycle. If her menstruation does not already align with the moon, she will connect to it twice a month. However, once women begin aligning their energy with herbs, practices, and lifestyle choices to flow with the regenerative currents of nature, the menstrual cycle often will align, and they will begin to bleed either on the full or dark moon. Some say that bleeding with the dark moon means you are in a "mother phase" of life, and bleeding with the full moon signifies you are in a "priestess phase." Many women will bleed with either the dark or full moon and then switch every few months, depending on the energetics and transformations occurring in their personal and creative lives.

Tracking your menstrual cycle and how you feel throughout the lunar cycle is a wonderful way to learn directly from the magickal alchemy of your body, life, and connection to Nature. Each of us is a unique being undergoing continual transformations. Learning from our own experience helps us journey with greater awareness as we cycle around the wheel of the year, spiraling, never finding ourselves in the exact same space, given the third dimension of time.

For those who are not bleeding, resting with the dark moon and adopting the practices of this portal also allows you to enter the magickal energies where the veil is thin. It is a psychic time, ideal for divination, shamanic journeying, meditation, and the spiritual renewal that is found in the fertile void.

The practice of resting on the night of the new moon extends to our gardens as well. In biodynamic agriculture, we never do any gardening on the new moon. It is considered a day to rest, an important practice to cultivate regeneration in the Earth.

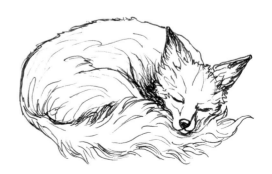

BLEEDING INTO THE EARTH

Our whole and holy bodies shed sacred blood. As we reclaim our tools as Witches, we reclaim our bodies as holy, as one of our greatest vehicles connecting us to the sacred. Part of this means healing our personal and collective trauma around menstruation. For ages, stories have been created about the "impurity" of women's blood, but in fact—or perhaps because—our blood mysteries are a great source of power. Our cycles move like the moon, in twenty-eight-day cycles. When we bleed, we shed ourselves.

Bleed into the Earth, sisters, whenever possible. The status quo is to bleed into tampons or pads with bleach and chemicals on them. Let us change the status quo. Collect your blood in a menstrual cup, sea sponge, cloth, or period panties, wring it out in a bowl of water to dilute it, and give it to the plants and soil. Your blood makes amazing, mineral-rich plant food. We have the ability to give ourselves to the earth. I have heard legends spoken that the Earth needs blood for balance—as a gardener, I understand this point—and that when women begin giving their blood back to the Earth again, balance will be restored and men will stop shedding their blood in warfare. It may be a legend, or it may be a truth woven into the Great Mystery. It is certainly worth trying. And for the sacred self, the magick of this rite is deeply felt.

THE FIRST SPARK OF IMBOLC: PREGNANT IN THE VOID OF GAIA'S DEEP DREAM

The cross-quarter holy day of Imbolc (February 1 or 2) is celebrated as the midpoint between Winter Solstice and Spring Equinox. It marks the first stirring of the flame within. Imbolc connects us to the seed inside the fertile void of darkness. The seed will grow and sprout in the Spring—new creations, projects, and dreams will burst through us at that time. At Imbolc, it is still too soon to know what form they will take. Nonetheless, we begin to feel that something is coming. We connect to the spirit of the seed inside of us. This is the start of energy that will only continue to grow and blossom as we rebirth ourselves and begin to ride the waxing currents of energy into the portals of Spring.

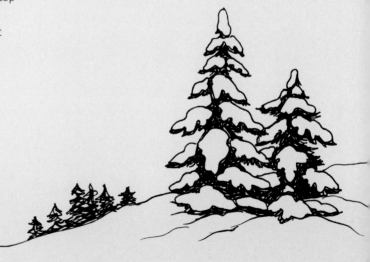

The Crone Archetype

The Crone is the hermit, the hag, the old lone wolf in a cave. She may be mad or enlightened—it is not for us to know. She is like Baba Yaga; she lives alone. Many fear her, yet she is the one we seek when we are lost in the dark. She is the one who lives closest to the void, so there are some mysterious similarities between the crone and the newborn. In many traditional cultures, the elders and the newborns spend much time together. Today, research shows how mutually beneficial this relationship is.

In our modern culture, our lives extend, and thus this portal holds a range of experiences. Many people in their seventies are incredibly youthful and engaged with community; many still work.

When working with archetypes, our true age does not matter. We enter the portal of the North in order to practice dissolving into void consciousness. We take time alone in order to renew ourselves. We journey into the mysteries with shamanic practices in order to grow and heal in all realms and worlds.

Opposite the Mother archetype on the wheel, the Crone brings balance to our culture, which pushes perpetual Summer and doing. We have much work to do in the realms of unraveling, unwinding, dropping deeper, and dissolving our egos into the velvet folds of the fertile void.

From there we came and to there we will return. The less afraid we are of the Crone, the more familiar we become with the threshold of darkness, and the more we can regenerate ourselves and our world.

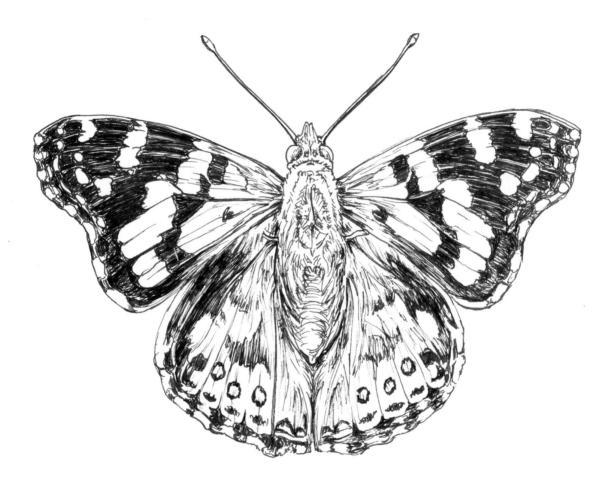

Earth Medicine of the North: Entering the Void and Restorative Rest

As all of Nature sleeps and dissolves into the darkness of Winter's renewal, so too you may ask for the plants to help you journey into other realms and into deep restorative rest.

What we began in the Fall allows us to enter void consciousness and the portal of renewal. The consciousness shifting plants and nervines we worked with as the energy of the year waned in the Fall months helped us release the worldly doings of the Summer so that we could travel lightly into the darkening months and Winter Solstice. Our meditation practices deepened, and our ability to be calm and still prepared us for the wisdom years of the Crone. In the Winter months, we continue to work with nervines and sedatives to bring silence into the nervous system. By frequently entering a meditative state, we can learn to become masters of our nervous systems, which is where our greatest power as Witches and humans is found. Rather than reacting unconsciously to our triggers and emotions, we learn to broaden our perspectives and witness our nervous systems as mechanisms of connection and communication, not allowing them to be the rulers of our beings. As we bring balance to the mind with nervines and deepen our meditation practice, we also continue to strengthen the nervous system with adaptogens.

Adaptogens are some of the oldest tonic herbs of our planet, plants that have adapted to thrive in various conditions over many thousands of years. They are resilient and hardy, and they hold deep vigor. They connect us to some of the most ancient traditions of medicine in the various cultures that have held them. Ginseng, reishi, chaga, rhodiola, eleuthero, schisandra, nettles, gotu kola, and ashwagandha are examples of adaptogens that ancestors of different lands have used

as longevity tonics. They help us age gracefully as they tone the mind, strengthen the nervous system and heart, and support circulation, digestion, immunity, and all processes in the body. Some, such as reishi, are said in traditional Chinese medicine to be shen tonics—strengthening the wisdom of the spirit. Indeed, all these plants have evolved and seen significant changes on our planet. When we work with them consistently, they make us more adaptable and resilient. Adaptogens replenish our deep roots, helping us access greater vitality, strength, vigor, and health. Some adaptogens are roots, and some are mushrooms. Both groups are connected to the darkness of the Earth and help us journey down into the dark realms of mystery.

Medicinal mushrooms are both adaptogenic and powerful spiritual helpers in weaving us into the intelligence of the Earth, the Web of Life, and the mysterious soil, where plants converse and exchange energy via the fungal and mycelial network. Winter is my favorite time to meditate with the spirit of reishi. The initial nervine action silences my busy human mind, grounds my energy, and helps me arrive in a meditative state of silence and stillness. As I invite the spirit of reishi in and continue to sip my infusion during the meditation, I begin to journey into the fertile darkness, which connects the realms of Below and Above. I feel my third eye open and my mind expand, while my circulation increases and energy moves in my brain. I then bring in my intention and work to rewire my brain, to weave myself into the larger fabric of the universe.

Meditating with plants is truly the greatest source of wisdom, expansion, and teachings for me. Psychotropic plants, such as "magick mushrooms," ayahuasca, peyote, and San Pedro, are widely acknowledged as teacher plants. However, in the Wise Woman tradition of restorative and nutritive medicine, we acknowledge that *all* plants are teacher plants. All plants can shift our consciousness. After all, inviting another energy and spirit into our bodies to connect with our essence will shift us, connecting us to the alchemy of the connection in unfoldment. That said, psychotropic shamanic plants are connected to the gateway of the North. They help us enter other realms beyond the three-dimensional existence governed by the laws of time and space. When administered in sacred space and ceremony by a real shaman and holder of a lineage, great healing to the spirit may occur.

These plants are very powerful: just look at the current scientific evidence supporting microdosing with psilocybin to help rewire the brain, with significant results for those struggling with depression. But as some of them become more popular, be aware that they are being shared irresponsibly, and there is risk of serious harm in those situations. Make sure you are grounded in yourself when seeking to expand outside of yourself.

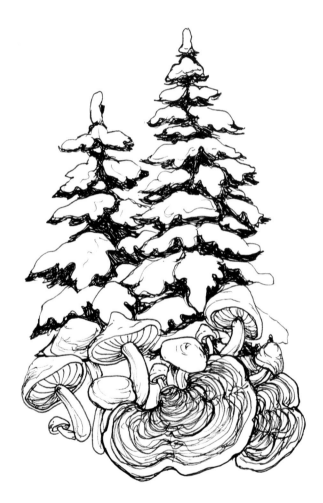

SANTA CLAUS WAS A SHAMAN
DRESSED LIKE A HALLUCINOGENIC MUSHROOM

As we unearth the pagan roots of our cultural traditions, we learn more about the rituals that we perform and their significance. Christmas, the Christian holiday celebrating the birth of Christ, is celebrated just after Winter Solstice, when the sun/son/God is born anew. Long ago, in Nordic European lands, people would spend time snowed into their huts, moving as little as possible to conserve energy and food—probably meditating, hibernating, sleeping, telling stories, and sharing dreams and visions. Stories say that in Northern Europe, shamans and holders of *Amanita muscaria*, or flying mushroom, would travel with their reindeer sleds, climb in through chimneys (because folks were snowed in), and bring the "gift of Christmas"—hallucinogenic mushroom tea. These mushrooms naturally grow under fir trees, popping up like the surprise gifts we place under our Christmas trees. The evergreen trees of fir and pine represent eternal life. At a time when not much in nature was showing signs of life, people would decorate their homes with evergreens. I have heard that our tradition of decorating the evergreen trees comes from hanging the red and white mushrooms to dry on the tree. The traveling carriers of the mushroom medicine would also decorate themselves with fir and wear the red and white colors of the flying mushroom. Perhaps Santa and his flying reindeer once brought the gift of shamanic journeys and expansion of the mind in the time of darkness.

As above, so below. When we enter the portal of the dark moon, the pause between breaths, the fertile void, we connect to the mirrored realms of the microcosm and macrocosm. If we journey shamanically into the realms below, perhaps by meditating with a mushroom such as reishi, we often end up arriving in the realms above, the starry places and the invisible web of communication that our upper chakras open us to. Above and below connect, as do the inbreath and outbreath and the waning energy of Nature and her waxing rebirth.

The Crone aspect journeys shamanically, gathering medicine and working healing in other realms. She balances this with getting deep, restorative rest in the realm beyond dreaming, where there is no conscious awareness. The hibernating animals of Winter model the medicine of Winter, and we work with sedatives to enter deep sleep. The slowest brain waves human produce fall in the delta range of 0.5 to 4 Hertz. They can be difficult for adults to access—nearly impossible for most during the waking state and sometimes even difficult if sleep is disturbed or light. These are the most regenerative brain waves, corresponding with which the body repairs and heals itself and produces the human growth hormone. Sedating herbs such as hops, valerian, kava kava, and poppy help us enter deep states of sleep, in which our bodies heal and restore healthy functions and from which we emerge renewed.

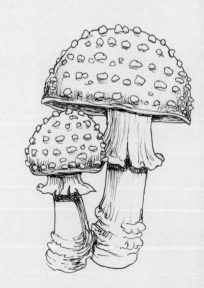

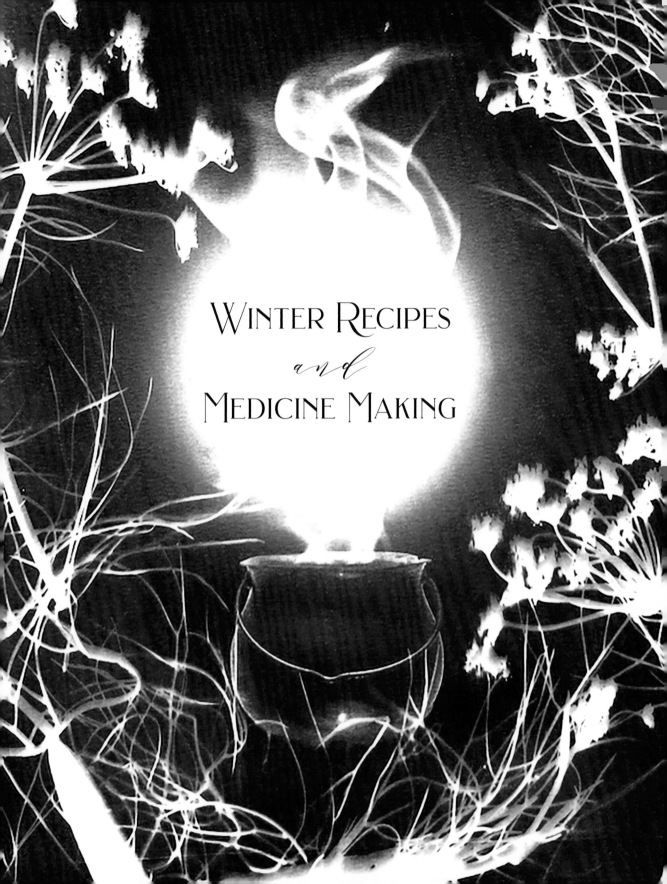

Winter Recipes
and
Medicine Making

Blessing Herbs

Winter is the perfect time to weave blessing herbs into your apothecary when the cold winter strengthens the aromatic oils of evergreens and our spirits journey with sacred smokes into the darkness of the night. Burning blessing herbs at the new moon is also magickal for helping us enter the portal of the North. Read about blessing herbs and sacred smokes on pages 30 to 31 and spend your Winter gathering local evergreen needles.

In this season, juniper, cedar, and pine are all in their peak of aromatic medicine. You may find pine resin on a pine cone; if you do not live in a snowy climate, search the base of an evergreen tree by brushing your fingertips on the Earth around the trunk, and you will likely find little tears of resin that you collect and burn on a charcoal. Never harvest resin directly from a tree, as it is then being used for protection and healing by the tree.

Pine Oil

Pine oil is such a magickal oil that is easy to make in abundance and is utterly divine. Whenever I smell pine oil, I think of Sage Maurer, who taught me how to make it and who pours copious amounts of the beautiful oils she makes from her land into hot baths—an evergreen queen. Not only is a hot bath with pine oil deeply relaxing and grounding, it also opens the heart and respiratory system, calms the mind, and centers us in an open heart. It is a wonderful oil to use if you are sick with a cold or flu.

Fill a large jar with pine needles. You may use scissors to trim the needles into 1- or 2-inch (2.5 to 5 cm) pieces to release the oils, or place them in a blender and cover with olive oil, blend, and then pour into your jar. Olive oil is a wonderfully thick oil that is deeply penetrating and nutritive to the skin as well as inexpensive, so you can make a lot and use often. Let your pine oil infuse for eight months or more, shaking every once in a while, then strain. Use as a massage oil or foot oil, or pour into a hot bath for the most blissful experience.

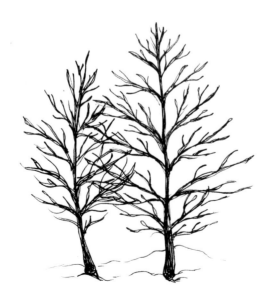

Sweet Dreams Tea

This tea is wonderfully relaxing; I formulated it for a woman struggling with insomnia. It has sedative herbs that help support a full night's sleep, nervines that calm the mind, and plants that comfort the heart and spirit. The stevia leaf and licorice root give it a pleasantly sweet and aromatic flavor without the artificial taste that stevia extracts often have.

Yield: 2¼ cups (164 g)

3 tablespoons (13.5 g) hops
2 tablespoons (4 g) lemon balm
3 tablespoons (15 g) passion vine
3 tablespoons (5 g) linden leaf and flower
2 tablespoons (4 g) motherwort
2 tablespoons (24 g) licorice root
3 tablespoons (17 g) oat straw
2 tablespoons (14 g) eleuthero root
3 tablespoons (14 g) chamomile flowers
2 tablespoons (15 g) valerian root
3 tablespoons (14 g) California poppy
3 tablespoons (14 g) skullcap
2 tablespoons (3 g) holy basil
2 tablespoons (7 g) stevia leaf

1. Blend the herbs together in a bowl and transfer to store in a jar, using a handful in a quart size jar of hot water or filing a tea strainer to make an infusion of 20 minutes or more each evening to take you into sweet dreams.

Sweetly Rooted I Rise Tea

This tea blend draws on the grounding, adaptogenic, nourishing properties of medicinal roots similar to the Sweet, Spicy, Alive, and Awake Tea blend found in the Spring portal (page 69). This blend is more calming, less activating, with a stronger descending energy from the roots and lymph-drainage herbs. This blend can help us nourish the deep roots of winter while warming our hearts and bones, grounding us and calming the nervous system.

Sometimes the energies of Winter have enough of a strong gravitational pull. If you need to balance the slowness and depth of the Winter portal with something more activating and enlivening, I recommend drinking the spicier Spring version. That version also helps us with digestion, which can sometimes get bogged down and too slow in the Winter months. Ask your body what would feel most nourishing.

Yield: ½ cup (50 g)

1 tablespoon (7 g) eleuthero root
1 tablespoon (7 g) burdock root
1 tablespoon (7 g) dandelion root
2 tablespoons (14 g) astragalus root
1 tablespoon (7 g) marshmallow root
1 tablespoon (3.75 g) Ceylon cinnamon chips
¼ teaspoon (2 g) licorice root
¼ teaspoon (2 g) ginger root (optional)

1. Combine all ingredients and store in an airtight container.

2. Use one handful of the blend per quart (946 ml) of water. Either make a hot overnight infusion or simmer gently, covered, on the stove for at least 30 minutes. Add more water as necessary.

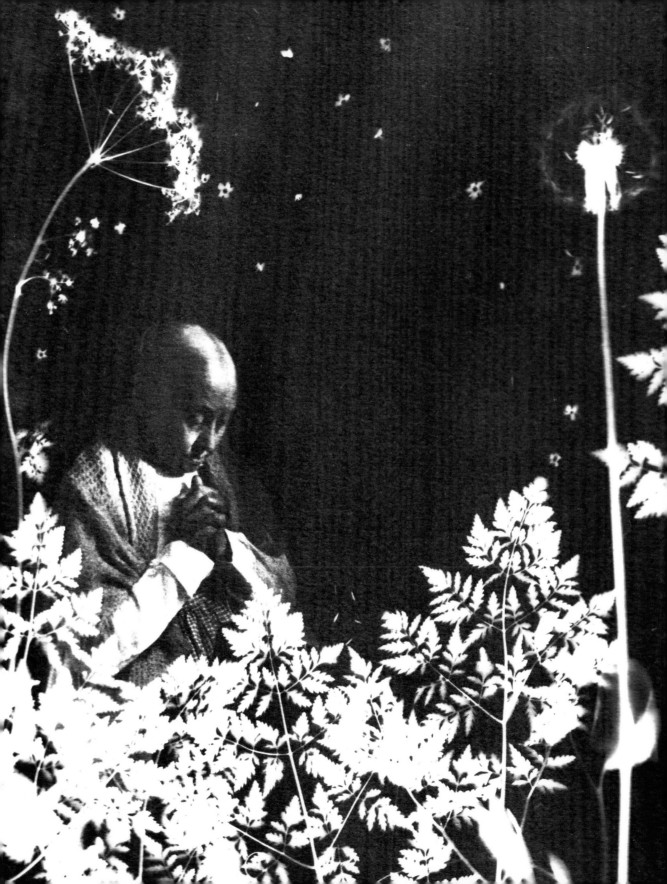

In the Garden, on the Earth

Nature sleeps. The plants have died back. Their life force is in their roots, in the dark, dreaming Earth. A blanket of snow covers them, and they come into stillness, dissolving their consciousness into the silent song of Winter, of humming mycelia, of frozen stillness. This portal is the pause in between breaths, from which comes renewal.

Let your garden rest. If you live in snowy climates, prepare for the Winter by putting it to sleep. In the Fall, cut back dead brush. For the Winter, you may cover your soil with mulch, leaf litter, or a cover crop to protect the Earth and life below.

Enjoy the songs of silence and the hum of dreams in the wildness. With snowshoes, you can walk on water above feet of dreaming shrubs and branches. Follow your intuition and guide yourself on paths between trees that you would never be able to traverse when the land is growing and the bushes are thick, taking any path you wish, or one that does not exist, thus embodying the movements of a sovereign Crone. This is the time of exploring unknown realms, both inside and outside yourself.

In climates where there is no snow, learn to love the look of death. Maybe the wilderness is brown and dry, or maybe it's wet and rainy. Practice solitude in your walking meditations and gaze love onto the dreaming Earth. How freeing it is to be like a Crone, unattached to looking nice for others. Find the beauty in dead things, in unkept wilderness, in places left behind as the attention of Gaia journeys into the mysteries of the roots and dark realms below.

During the seasons of Fall and Winter, the energy of the Earth goes inward, and the plants draw their energy into their roots, go dormant, or die back. This is the inbreath of our planet, mirrored in the evening of each twenty-four-hour cycle. The inbreath energy is a good time to prune, nourish the soil, and spread compost. When it's time to enter the North's portal through the dark moon, we allow our gardens to rest.

When I die, let me be the most delicious cosmic compost for the Earth!

I see the stars in my bones returning into the darkness of her microcosmic soil flesh. One day, I will be good food.

For now, I will continue digesting the currents from the heavens and Earth, making myself delicious.

Winter Rituals and Self-Care

Winter is a time to do nothing—to do no thing. This can be very challenging to the modern human. The rituals and self-care of Winter are simple and spacious, so you can follow the lack of linear instruction into nonlinear realms of deep healing and magick. Discover what helps you deeply unwind. Go back to rituals of release if cords entangle in a capitalistic push of productivity connected to self-worth. See how deep you can go with less. Discover the mysteries and magick that await.

Herbal Sauna

In the coldness of Winter, saunas support circulation and warm us to our core. If you have access to a dry sauna, consider bringing in aromatic herbs such as eucalyptus, pine, birch, the evergreens, mugwort, or rosemary into it with you. Alternatively, boil branches in a big pot with a lid on so the steam does not evaporate, making a strong tea of aromatic clippings. Add to a hot bathtub and soak with the plants.

Sound Baths

Sound vibration can shift our brain waves into the theta and delta brain waves that are associated with deeper states of consciousness and restorative rest. Find a sound bath near you, and bring a blanket and eye pillow. Crystal bowls, tuning forks, and gongs emanate different frequencies, which can bring us into deep states of meditation and relaxation.

Pink Himalayan Salt Lamps

I highly recommend using pink Himalayan salt lamps in your home, especially in the evenings, to shift you into restorative realms. Blue light from electronics disrupts melatonin and sleep hormones and can lead to insomnia or shallow sleep. In addition to creating a soothing, warm, and beautiful light, salt lamps purify the air, neutralize electromagnetic radiation, and generate negative ions, thus improving air quality, treating seasonal affective disorder, enhancing mood and relaxation, and improving sleep.

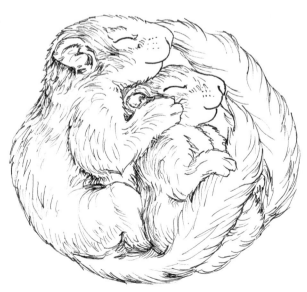

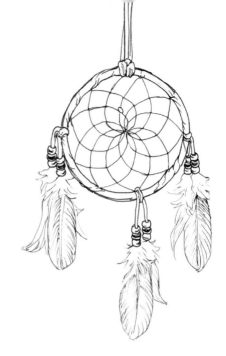

Be a Cat

If you have a cat, you can learn what restorative rest looks like by observing the luxuriation of naps on the floor where a beam of light hits. Be a cat. For hours.

Observe a Day of Silence

Take a day of silence. You will likely have to mark this day weeks in advance, planning accordingly and letting loved ones know. Make a little name tag that says, "Today I am in silence :)" Point to it and smile if people talk to you.

Wake up without saying a word and go to sleep that day not having used your voice. Don't answer text messages, read or write emails, or read books. Have you ever done this before? I won't tell you what will happen, but I will tell you it is magickal, revealing, healing, and deeply restorative.

Sleep with Moonlight and Darkness

People are becoming more aware of the importance of deep sleep for their health and productivity, so you may start seeing many shared resources on how to "hack" your sleep. If you have trouble staying asleep, it is worth following some of these dietary and lifestyle recommendations. The Witch's preferred method for supporting a healthy sleep cycle is to sleep in complete darkness, with no electronic lights, and near a window through which the natural light of the moon and rising sun may shine. If you live in a city, however, I do recommend a blackout curtain.

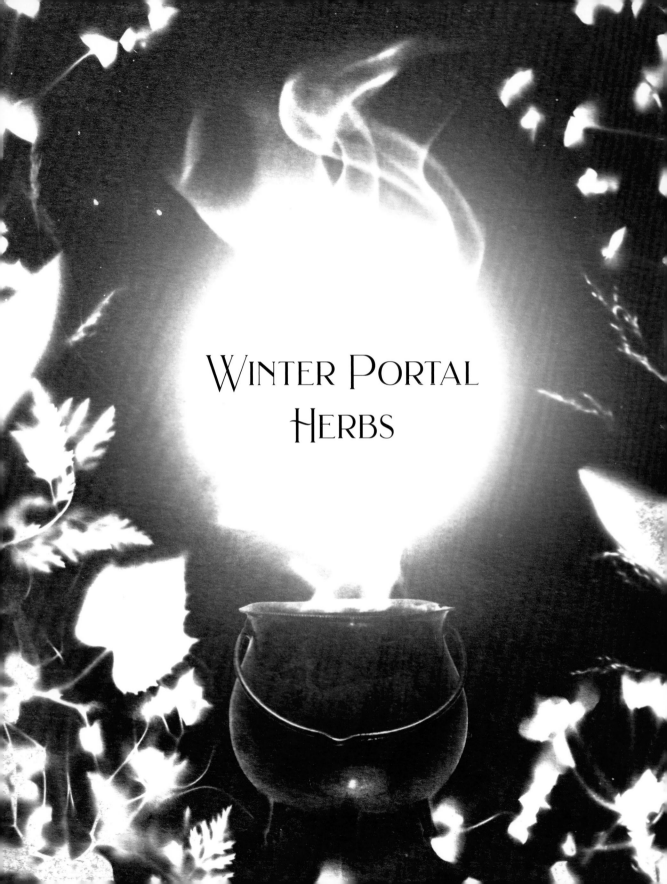

Winter Portal Herbs

plant profile

Hops

LATIN NAME *Humulus lupulus*

FAMILY Cannabaceae (hemp family)

A tall perennial clinging, flowering vine with green-yellow catkins and heart-shaped, serrated leaves. Hops are native to Europe but grow in western Asia and North America as well. Famous as an ingredient in beer, its sedative properties have been woven into folk medicine and lore for centuries.

HERBAL AND MEDICINAL PROPERTIES

- Strong nervine and sedative: an ally that helps us deeply relax and enter restorative sleep and full-body relaxation

- Antispasmodic: relieves cramps and melts tension from the body

- Aromatic bitter: supports digestion and healing to ulcers and IBS

- Externally healing to skin infections

PLANT SPIRIT HEALING

Hops sedate and bring us into deep silence. When I meditate with hops, I usually have to lie down. This plant allows us to relax the body and mind, showing us how deeply tired we may be. Hops open the portals to deep, uninterrupted rest and make it a priority. A wonderful ally for insomniacs or people with severe anxiety or who can't stop "doing."

FAVORITE USES

- Tincture for treating sleeplessness, anxiety, or panic attacks

- Tea with honey for sleep.

- As part of Sweet Dreams Tea (see page 201)

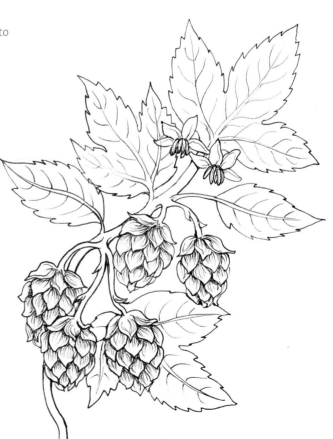

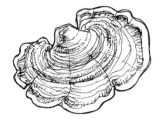

plant profile
Reishi

LATIN NAME *Ganoderma lucidum*

FAMILY Ganodermataceae

This shiny, red-varnished, kidney-shaped, flat polypore mushroom grows on trees and decaying trunks in Asian and North American forests and is cultivated on logs. It has no gills on the underside, releasing its spores through fine pores that are generally cream colored. It is a prized ancient herb of traditional Chinese medicine and is one of the oldest mushrooms with written records of medicinal use—dating back over two thousand years. Its Chinese name, *lingzhi*, means miraculous, sacred, divine, mysterious, or effective mushroom of longevity.

HERBAL AND MEDICINAL PROPERTIES

- Longevity herb, adaptogen: considered an elixir of life and plant of immortality; strengthens our ability to resist stressors, increasing health, vitality, stamina, mental clarity
- Shen tonic: develops wisdom and spirit; used by Taoist monks to increase health and vitality and to facilitate spiritual experiences
- Immunomodulator: has the intelligence, discernment, and ability to balance an overactive and suppressed immune system; as such, and with antiviral properties, it is an ally for chronic viral infections and HIV
- Antibacterial, antitumor properties: supportive in healing from cancer; protective in conjunction with other cancer treatments
- Protective to DNA, antioxidant rich, and anti-inflammatory
- Heart tonic, hepatoprotector: strengthening to the cardiovascular system, balancing to blood sugars, lowers cholesterol
- Cleansing to the body; balancing to the heart, brain, and mind

PLANT SPIRIT HEALING

As a mushroom, reishi brings the magick of the stars and void consciousness into the dark soil, composting places, and dreaming Earth. When I meditate with mushroom, I am brought to the invisible network of connection that weaves from my body into the Earth and from my brain into the night sky of the cosmos. Regardless of whether I journey up or down, I end up in the cosmic void. The spirit of reishi weaves us into the supreme intelligence and mystery of the Great Web of Life. There, we can meditate and access deep states of consciousness while our physical body receives the calming and grounding properties of the plant's medicine. A powerful ally to rebalance our nervous system and help our minds and vibrations evolve, reishi is said to help clear karma. I understand karma as something we create when we react to unconscious triggers and wounds. (I thank my friend Larry Novick, a shaman and therapist, for this definition of karma.) There are many plants—reishi, tulsi, and kava kava, included—that bring us into higher states of consciousness, which our nervous system can learn to hold and attune to with practice. I believe this may be similar instruction to what Taoist monks received in their meditations: as we attune ourselves to these wisdom plants, our consciousness evolves and we are less likely to fall into unconscious reaction to our vulnerabilities and wounds. Rather, we can learn to master our nervous system and respond with grace and in harmony.

FAVORITE USES

- Double extraction, in elixirs or diluted in water
- Decocted overnight as a tea or in broths, soups, herbal black coffee, and other recipes
- Hot overnight infusion
- Meditation with the infusion
- Placed on altars

Mugwort

LATIN NAME *Artemisia vulgaris*

FAMILY Asteraceae/Compositae (aster family)

Mugwort is found in temperate regions of the Northern Hemisphere. It flourishes in open areas and along roads and is gathered in late Summer just before flowering. A witchy perennial shrubby herb of the woods and stream banks, mugwort has a fuzzy silver underside to her thin, deeply toothed 4-inch (10 cm) leaves and grows about waist high. The flowers are tiny, blooming in the later Summer months. Leaves are best just before flowering; stems and dried herb are harvested after flowering for moxa sticks in acupuncture. Mugwort has a long history of lore. A magickal plant of dreaming and divination, as her name implies, she is associated with the moon goddess and has been used in the folk medicine of many traditions, especially as an ally to women and Witches.

HERBAL AND MEDICINAL PROPERTIES:

- Bitter digestive tonic: promotes digestion, production of bile, and enzymes
- Emmenagogue: encourages the shedding of the uterine wall and regulates menstruation; an ally to drink or steam vaginally to bring on menses; assists in full moon blood release; good for PMS and menopause
- Third eye opener, stimulating nervine: plant for divination and dreams, a consciousness shifter
- Antispasmodic: relaxing to cramps and tension in the body
- Dream herb: sleep with her for active dreams and astral travel, but do not expect a night of good rest

PLANT SPIRIT HEALING

Crone spirit, bitter, wise and true, mugwort pierces the veils of illusion, connecting us to unvarnished truth, while calming the body and nerves so we can go deep, unafraid of the mysteries. Stimulating to the womb, menses,

and sacral chakra, she can be called on to bring wisdom, perspective, and guidance to our creative endeavors. Because she's opening to the third eye, I often ask her to take me to places in my consciousness where my old ways are ready to be released. Work with her shamanically to balance the right and left hemispheres of the brain to bring in more magick from nonlinear realms, and to bend the laws of time and space. She's an herb for protection in magick, so you may carry her with you. She is beautiful and powerful in all her phases of growth, even when she has died back in Winter; her dry brown leaves retain their volatile oils and can be used for sacred smoke, blessing herbs, and moxa.

FAVORITE USES

- Tea as digestive bitter
- Sweetened tea for dreaming
- Sleep with her in the bed for astral travel
- Dried leaves and stems as kindling for starting a fire in the wild
- Shamanic journeying
- Herbal bathing and saunas
- To bring on menses, in a yoni steam, cleansing the womb

PRECAUTIONS

Avoid if pregnant.

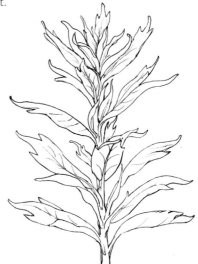

plant profile
Comfrey

LATIN NAME *Symphytum officinale*

FAMILY Boraginaceae (borage family)

Comfrey is a beloved perennial plant with large green leaves, hollow watery stems, and spiraling sacred purple bell flowers. A lover of watery places and moist soils, she is native to most of North America, Europe, and western Siberia and grows up to 3 feet (0.9 m) tall, spreading wide, especially if her roots are broken or disturbed. An ancient folk remedy, ally of witches and regenerative currents, comfrey is also called "bone knit," as she weaves magick into the mundane and is a powerful healer to injuries, tissues, skin, and wounds. Both root and leaves are used.

HERBAL AND MEDICINAL PROPERTIES

- Vulnerary: a powerful wound healer That can be used topically as a poultice or salve in the case of a burn, scrape, cut or rash; it heals so quickly that if the cut is deep, it is advised not to apply it, because it will heal the surface skin layer faster than the membranes can heal deeper down in the cut; comfrey salve is my go-to for all burns, skin rashes, scars, broken bones, sprained tendons, etc.
- Expectorant: comfrey's lung-shaped leaves and the tiny hairs covering the plant speak to its affinity for the respiratory system
- Demulcent: soothing to inflamed tissue; I drink comfrey juice or tea to heal inflammation or internal irritation caused by acid reflux, a bacterial infection, etc.
- Ally for regenerating the body and soul and starting a healing process and rebirth

PLANT SPIRIT HEALING

Beloved comfrey is my master teacher in times of death, rebirth, and regeneration. In one of the most difficult and traumatic times in my life, when my root chakra was suddenly severed, comfrey spoke to me in the garden and told me she would heal my root and help me grow new, more vital roots. And so it began, our journey together through the mysteries of life, a new chapter of my life beginning--indeed one where I was able to draw from much deeper reserves of Earth magick, nourishment, strength, and resilience. Comfrey is a master regenerator; if you try to dig her out of the garden, each place where you break the root will create life, to be reborn again. She's an ally during times of crisis, when we must allow old parts of ourselves to die and return to the Earth so we can be reborn. Healing to the soil, comfrey composts her leaves in unfurling waves, laying them like poultices on the body of the Earth, releasing deep nutrition into the soil. Use in compost piles and plant at the base of fruit trees; her deep taproots bring nutrition up and support the plants growing around her. While she deeply regenerates and heals our root chakras, she also nourishes us on a cellular level and opens the third eye and crown chakra, showing the golden ratio in her purple bell-shaped flowers that spiral open.

FAVORITE USES

- Fresh juice
- In herbal tea and blends with nourishing herbs
- As a healing poultice
- As a salve
- Flower essences
- In the garden, for compost, and in landscape design, planted in orchards
- Easy to propagate by placing a piece of the root in a pot of soil; delightful to gift

PRECAUTIONS

Comfrey has a bad reputation among some herbalists for containing small quantities of a toxic alkaloid, which can have a cumulative effect upon the liver. The largest concentrations are found in the roots; the leaves contain higher quantities of the alkaloid as they grow older, but young leaves contain almost none. Because of the wide range of stories from different herbalists, I work with comfrey when I need her magick, for up to a few days, with long breaks in between. I do not ingest her roots, working instead with mostly fresh, young leaves. I adore her but would not advise taking her daily for several months, especially if you have liver problems or are pregnant; otherwise I feel she is safe and her benefits have been profoundly healing for myself and others.

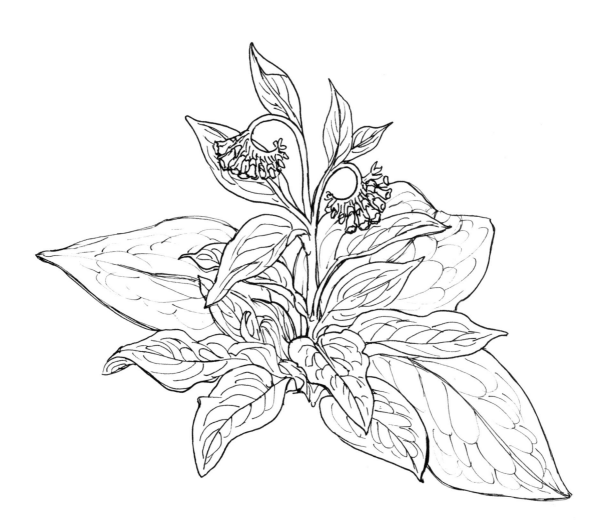

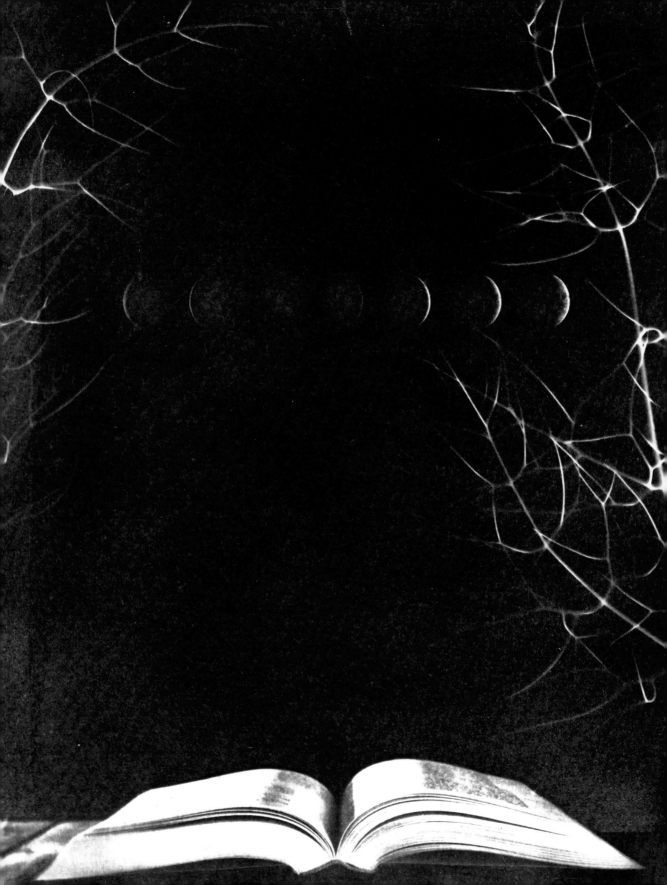

North Portal Journal Prompts

Reflect on the element of Earth in you.

Earth element in balance:

- Groundedness; caring for your environment, home, and body; ability to nourish yourself and create safety and support where needed

- Healthy root chakra, not carrying ancestral or family traumas, creating healing community

- Stability, reliability (balanced with fire)

- Healthy, good habits, mental calmness (balanced with air)

Earth element out of balance:

- Being overly emotional (too much water; usually needs earth or fire)

- Anxiety, panic attacks, being scattered mentally (needs more earth; air in chaos)

- Being stuck in your ways, stubborn, unyielding (too much earth; needs air to open your mind, fire or water to get unstuck, and an earth tonic that teaches how to hold earth in balance)

- Hoarding, overeating, accumulating (earth in chaos; needs fire to clear and transform radically, or water for more gentle, soft and emotion based releasing of layers. Earth tonics like nourishing herbs to balance the earth element.)

- Homelessness, unemployment, always changing jobs (needs more earth)

Reflect on how you can nourish your inner Crone archetype in your journal.

- If there were nothing I had to do, what would I do?

- What would I do differently if there were no social rules and no judgment?

- Am I tired? Am I resting enough?

- What would be the most divine rest for my body?

- What kind of rest does my heart desire?

- How does my mind want to rest?

- What is my dream refuge and retreat for my soul right now?

- How do I cultivate my inner Crone?

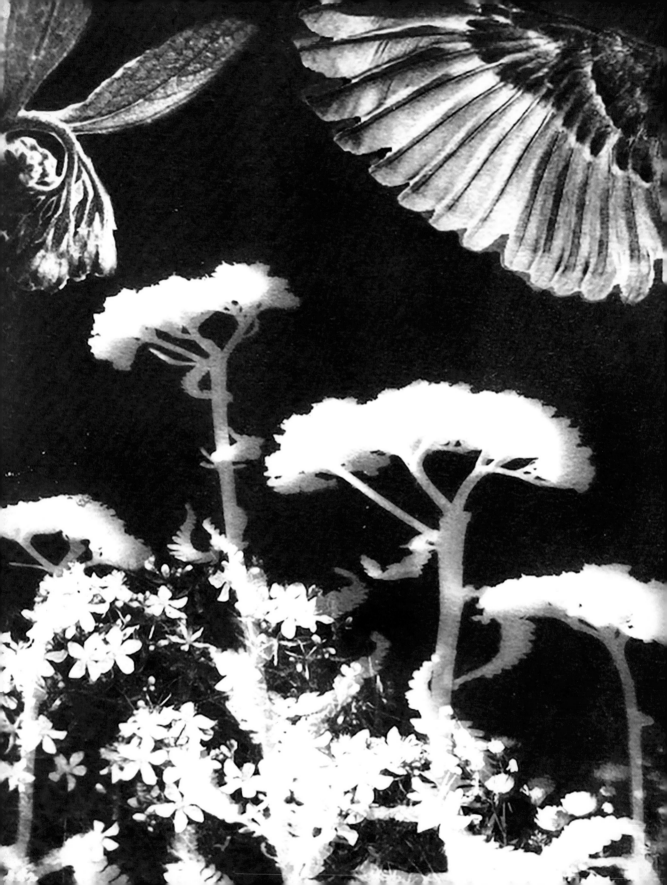

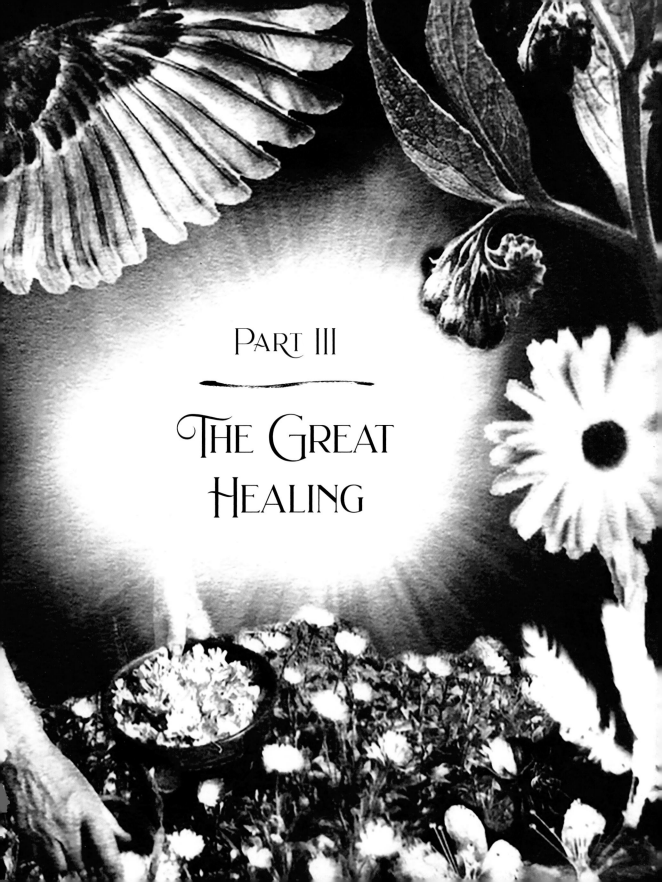

PART III

THE GREAT
HEALING

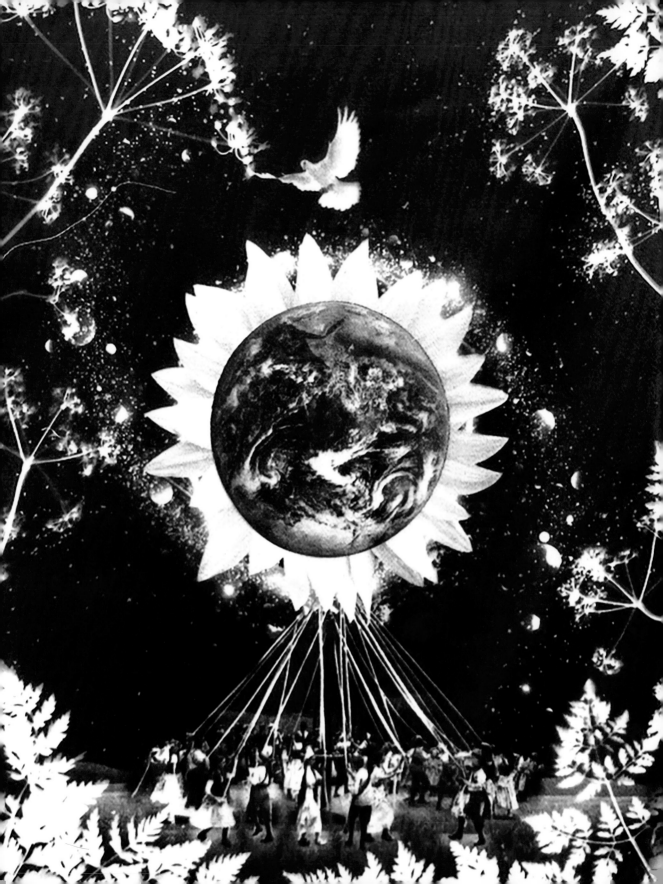

Chapter 8

Dancing the Spiral of Light

There are myths and prophecies that speak of the time we are in as a time of great transformation. Buddhist scholar and environmental activist Joanna Macy calls this time the Great Turning. She tells the stories of the Shambala warriors who go into the portals of darkness and illusion to bring light, healing, and transformation on behalf of the Great Turning—this is a prophecy of regeneration. Other ancient stories speak of people from all walks of life and cultures coming together as the rainbow warriors who will bring healing to our planet at a time of environmental devastation and ecological despair. In the Americas, we have the legends of the condor and eagle, who begin flying together, bringing us out of cultures of dominance and bringing our world back into balance.

I am a mother, a Witch, a lover of this Earth, and I am humble before the Great Mystery. I have hope for our future, for hope fuels my heart and actions and helps me make medicine of my life. For me, being hopeless and falling into despair would be a disservice to this web of magick, this tapestry we dance in. It would not feel right to speak projections of doom into the great unknown. In my heart, I feel the Great Web needs songs of beauty to be sung into the strings of creation—songs of love and faith. I imagine what the choir of our hopes strung together sound like. I can feel the harmonies, the unexpected delight of alchemical song. In the feeling, I affirm that *it is done*.

And so I sing my love song to the Earth. I work to create sanctuaries where my brothers and sisters can fall in love with the Earth, with themselves, and with the Great Mystery of Spirit.

May we love the Earth in deep devotion and great beauty.

Falling in Love with the Earth

Love is the greatest motivation, the greatest source of healing and miracles. Humans take responsibility for those they love.

As an educator, environmentalist, Green Witch, devotee of the Earth, mother, and lover, I see how creating opportunities for people to cultivate embodied relationship with the Earth opens their hearts and senses to the miracles of being alive, being a part of Gaia. When our hearts open to Nature, we heal and blossom. When we fall in love with the Earth, the unique gifts that are dormant in our souls and centers of action may awaken, and we may become embodied medicine.

It is easy to look at the conveniences of modern living, such as plastic or online shopping, and become discouraged in humanity. However, shame and guilt do not motivate our brothers and sisters into an open and long-lasting transformation of behavior. It is love that opens us up to feel the pain of the polluted oceans and the miracles of the womb from which all of life crawled out of.

Fall in Love with the Earth.
Fall in Love with yourself.
Be the most devoted lover to Her.
Sing songs and praise to the Great Mystery.
Make your life a magickal, radical act of Love, a living prayer.
Make beauty, make medicine, be medicine.
Be love,
spiraling out in ecstatic unfoldment.

Thank you.
May you be blessed.
And so it is.

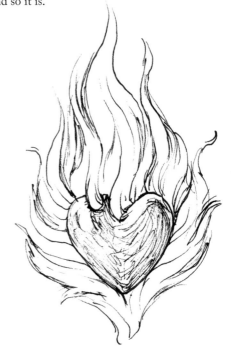

MOVING FORWARD AND AROUND AGAIN:
DANCING THE SPIRAL OF LIFE

"How deep will I take you?"
says the Great Mystery
"You know I've birthed galaxies, star child.
I am relentless, because you are devoted.
You've spoken vows into the cosmic womb and perhaps
I am calling you to be a cauldron of transformation
that transcends the limits of one small lifetime.
You work beyond the laws of time,
so let your body catch up and digest starlight like the trees.
The garden rich in death and decay is also effortlessly fertile.
There, barefoot and naked, we have always danced,
stretching each other in delightful discovery
humble play and awe,
tears, ecstasy, and prayers.

So drink the holy water.
Gather the flowers,
brush your daughters' hair.
You have lifetimes to transform and nothing else to do.
One may say there is great urgency,
but approach it always anchored in deep time.
For it's urgency that got us in this mess in the first place.
Yes, this is the cosmic joke—
you want to stretch the laws of time,
so time will stretch you first.
Then, we come back to the dance again.
I'll birth galaxies through you.
So stretch and empty.
Eat the stars.
Dance the cosmos into being through your hips.
We are all born with this rite.
Remember?

RESOURCES

World as Lover, World as Self: Courage for Global Justice and Ecological Renewal by Joanna Macy

Plant Spirit Medicine: A Journey into Healing Wisdom of Plants by Eliot Cowan

The Garden Awakening: Designs to Nurture our Land and Ourselves by Mary Reynolds

Working the Roots: Over 400 Years of Traditional African American Healing by Michele Elizabeth E. Lee

Farming While Black: Soul Fire Farm's Practical Guide to Liberation on the Land by Leah Penniman

Permaculture Design: A Step-by-Step Guide by Aranya

The Practice of Traditional Western Herbalism: Basic Doctrine, Energetics, and Classification by Matthew Wood

Forgotten Fires: Native Americans and the Transient Wilderness by Omer C. Stewart

The Hidden Life of Trees: What They Feel, How They Communicate—Discoveries from a Secret World by Peter Wohlleben

Tending the Wild: Native American Knowledge and the Management of California's Natural Resources by M. Kat Anderson

Braiding Sweetgrass: Indigenous Wisdom, Scientific Knowledge, and the Teachings of Plants by Robin Wall Kimmerer

The Gift of Healing Herbs: Plant Medicines and Home Remedies for a Vibrantly Healthy Life by Robin Rose Bennett

Eastern Body, Western Mind: Psychology and the Chakra System as a Path to the Self by Anodea Judith

Cunt: A Declaration of Independence by Inga Muscio

Women Who Run with the Wolves: Myths and Stories of the Wild Woman Archetype by Clarissa Pinkola Estes

Biodynamic Gardening: Grow Healthy Plants and Amazing Produce with the Help of the Moon and Nature's Cycles by Monty Waldin

BIBLIOGRAPHY

Buhner, S. *Herbal Antibiotics: Natural Alternatives for Treating Drug-Resistant Bacteria*. Storey Publishing, 1999.

Buhner, S. *Herbal Antivirals: Natural Remedies for Emerging & Resistant Viral Infections*. Storey Publishing, 2013.

Dashu, Max. *Witches and Pagans: Women in European Folk Religion, 700–1100 (Secret History of the Witches)*. Veleda Press, 2017.

Hoffman, David. *Medicinal Herbalism: The Science and Practice of Herbal Medicine*. Healing Arts Press, 2003.

Holmes, Peter. *The Energetics of Western Herbs: A Materia Medica Integrating Western & Chinese Herbal Therapeutics*. Snow Lotus Press, 2007.

Maimes, S. and Winston, D. *Adaptogens: Herbs for Strength, Stamina and Stress Relief*. Healing Arts Press, 2007.

Mollison, B. and Slay R. *Introduction to Permaculture*. Ten Speed Press, 1997.

Starhawk. *The Spiral Dance: A Rebirth of the Ancient Religion of the Great Goddess*. HarperOne, 1999.

Steiner, Rudolf. *Agriculture Course: The Birth of the Biodynamic Method*. Rudolf Steiner Press, 2004.

Tedlock, Barbara. *The Woman in the Shaman's Body: Reclaiming the Feminine in Religion and Medicine*. Bantam Books, 2005.

Weed, Susan S. *Wise Woman Herbal: Healing Wise*. Ash Tree Publishing, 2003.

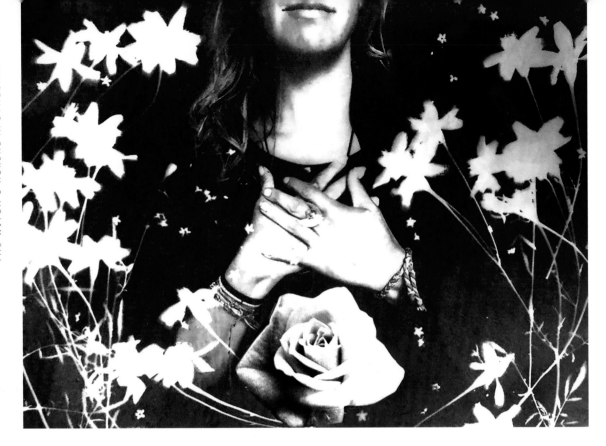

About the Author

Marysia Miernowska is an herbalist, Witch, and gardener rooted in the Wise Woman Tradition of Healing. She directs the California branch of the Gaia School of Healing and Earth Education, where she holds ceremony and teaches herbal medicine, plant shamanism, regenerative farming practice, and Earth magick. A multilingual and multicultural devotee of Mother Earth, Marysia has grown up internationally and traveled extensively, learning different ways of tending to the Earth and sharing regenerative, grassroots Earth medicine. She draws on her background as a community organizer and activist, and she keeps her feet rooted by designing and tending to medicinal gardens using permaculture and biodynamic practices. Marysia formulates herbal medicine, sees clients, and curates educational events at her apothecary, Wild Love Apothecary, in Topanga Canyon, California. She makes sacred plant botanicals for her community at her local apothecary and from the lands she tends, and also formulates and consults for other companies. She lives in Topanga, with her daughter Flora, grows herbs in Malibu, and teaches and holds ceremony in the greater Los Angeles area. She shares her passions with her students and community, in the gardens she tends and in her writing. You can follow Marysia on Instagram (@Marysia_Miernowska) and learn about the Sacred Plant Medicine Apprenticeship by visiting the Gaia School of Healing & Earth Education website (www.thegreenwoman.com).

This, Marysia's first book, is being released with a daily planner and a wall calendar to help guide you as you journey through the portals of time and transformation shared in this book. Visit thegaiaschoolofhealingcalifornia.com or wildloveapothecary.com for more information.

ᴀCKNOWLEDGEMENTS & GRATITUDES

I give gratitude to all the places, human and nonhuman midwives, and doulas who helped me bend the laws of time and space and birth this book.

Thank you to the human realms—my friends, allies, family, teachers, students, and Witches.

Thank you to Sage Maurer for caressing the pines open in the deep northern woods of Vermont and helping me see the green path that led me back to the nettles in my great-grandmother's hands and the linden trees of Poland. Words will never encompass the magick of who you are: teacher, sister, friend, ally, guide, poet, mystic, love. I am forever grateful for your generosity and friendship.

Thank you to my covens and the gardens I tend, land I love, Oak I teach under. Thank you Maggie Lochtenberg for your incredible work on the art for this book—I will forever delight in the trasmition and mutual delight of shared visions we caught from the ethers and that you so beautifully transcribed into the art that blesses these pages. Thank you to my many sistars who support me and my work and love me even though I work so much: Thank you Paula, Jade, Jesse, Valeria, and all my green Gaia witches whom I adore. Thank you to Jill for fishing this book from the deep waters of my being and the team of amazing women at The Quarto Group who made this book possible.

Thank you to the trees from whom this book is made. Please forgive me for any harm I have caused, for any beauty I write pales in comparison to yours. I do pray a miraculous force of love and magick ripples from these pages made of your body, awakening the wild hearts of readers and that currents of healing and devotion return to the lands from which you came and to the flesh of our Earth Mother. Thank you, siblings, for my daily breath and your participation.

Thank you to all that is invisible that partook in the birth of this book and the experiences that filled the wells of my being from which I draw healing nectars that I pray nourish thirsty or curious souls. The gratitudes to that which is unseen belongs in worlds beyond words.

I give gratitude to all the places and lands that held me as I stretched myself to write this. My sister Paula's hearth and the fire she tended where I began in the mountains of Yosemite on the Winter Solstice. The ridges and rocks I summited to ignite the channels of creation during the pregnant void of winter. Gratitude and reverence to the healing moonlit waters of hot springs and delighted otters that seduced the writing further after Imbolc. Thank you, Flora: I adore you, beloved daughter, miraculous spark, catalyst of transformation. You have changed me. Thank you, moja kochana córeczka. Gratitude to my mother and father, my chosen family, and my community who helped with Flora so I could squeeze in moments of writing. Blessings on my home where I labored into the nights of the Spring Equinox and blessings on my parents' home, where I read this one last time before releasing it in the night of the Solar Eclipse and July new moon. Deep bows to the reality of bending the laws of time and space, and all the unromantic moments of pushing a book out, afraid to share something so intimate and afraid of wavering in the fear of human judgment.

With gratitude to all the deaths and rebirths in my life that have fed my soul with flavors bitter and sweet. To the wholeness, ripeness, and complete mystery of life. All my devotion to our beautiful, beloved Earth Mother; to the plants, my teachers, healers, and guides. Thank you for all you have given me and taken away. One day, I will be the most delicious compost, exhaling songs of sweet decay into your fertile flesh. In the meantime, may I marry the soil and the stars in a great love song of my life. May my life be a living prayer that brings healing to those who have come before, and those who are yet unborn.

And so it is.

Marysia Miernowska

These gratitudes were cast on the other side of the lunar and solar Beltane portal
On a day it rained in May, in Topanga, California
With a black cat curled on my lap.

INDEX